Current Utilization of Biologicals

Editor

GREGORY S. KELLER

FACIAL PLASTIC SURGERY CLINICS OF NORTH AMERICA

www.facialplastic.theclinics.com

Consulting Editor
J. REGAN THOMAS

November 2018 • Volume 26 • Number 4

ELSEVIER

1600 John F. Kennedy Boulevard • Suite 1800 • Philadelphia, Pennsylvania, 19103-2899

http://www.theclinics.com

FACIAL PLASTIC SURGERY CLINICS OF NORTH AMERICA Volume 26, Number 4
November 2018 ISSN 1064-7406, ISBN-13: 978-0-323-64143-2

Editor: Jessica McCool
Developmental Editor: Sara Watkins

Facial Plastic Surgery Clinics of North America (ISSN 1064-7406) is published quarterly by Elsevier Inc., 360 Park Avenue South, New York, NY 10010-1710. Months of issue are February, May, August, and November. Business and Editorial Offices: 1600 John F. Kennedy Blvd., Suite 1800, Philadelphia, PA 19103-2899. Periodicals postage paid at New York, NY, and additional mailing offices. Subscription prices are $398.00 per year (US individuals), $628.00 per year (US institutions), $454.00 per year (Canadian individuals), $782.00 per year (Canadian institutions), $535.00 per year (foreign individuals), $782.00 per year (foreign institutions), $100.00 per year (US students), and $255.00 per year (foreign students). Foreign air speed delivery is included in all *Clinics* subscription prices. All prices are subject to change without notice. POSTMASTER: Send address changes to *Facial Plastic Surgery Clinics*, Elsevier Health Sciences Division, Subscription Customer Service, 3251 Riverport Lane, Maryland Heights, MO 63043. **Customer service: 1-800-654-2452 (US and Canada); 1-314-447-8871 (outside US and Canada); Fax: 314-447-8029; E-mail: journalscustomerservice-usa@elsevier.com (for print support); journalsonline support-usa@elsevier.com (for online support).**

Reprints. For copies of 100 or more of articles in this publication, please contact the Commercial Reprints Department, Elsevier Inc., 360 Park Avenue South, New York, NY 10010-1710. Tel.: 212-633-3874; Fax: 212-633-3820; E-mail: reprints@elsevier.com.

Facial Plastic Surgery Clinics of North America is covered in *MEDLINE/PubMed* (*Index Medicus*).

Contributors

CONSULTING EDITOR

J. REGAN THOMAS, MD
Professor, Facial Plastic and Reconstructive
Surgery, Department of Otolaryngology–Head
and Neck Surgery, Northwestern University
Feinberg School of Medicine, Chicago, Illinois,
USA

EDITOR

GREGORY S. KELLER, MD, FACS
Clinical Professor and Co-Director of the
Facial Plastic Surgery Fellowship, Department
of Head and Neck Surgery, Division of
Facial Plastic Surgery, David Geffen
School of Medicine, University of California,
Los Angeles, Los Angeles, USA; Attending
Physician, Cottage Hospital, Santa
Barbara, Santa Barbara, California,
USA

AUTHORS

KARAM W. BADRAN, MD
Division of Facial Plastic and Reconstructive
Surgery, Department of Head and Neck
Surgery, David Geffen School of Medicine,
University of California, Los Angeles,
Los Angeles, California, USA

LESLIE BAUMANN, MD, FAAD
Division of Cosmetic Dermatology, Founder,
University of Miami, Miami, Florida, USA

WILLIAM BEESON, MD
Facial Plastics, Clinical Professor,
Departments of Dermatology and
Otolaryngology–Head and Neck Surgery,
Indiana University School of Medicine,
Indianapolis, Indiana, USA

NATHAN BRYAN, PhD
Department of Molecular and Human Genetics,
Baylor College of Medicine, Houston, Texas,
USA

GREG CHERNOFF, BSc, MD, FRCS(C)
Chernoff Cosmetic Surgeons, Indianapolis,
Indiana, USA; Chernoff Cosmetic Surgeons,
Santa Rosa, California, USA; Chernoff
Cosmetic Surgeons, Xian, China

DIANE IRVINE DUNCAN, MD, FACS
Private Practice, Fort Collins, Colorado, USA

GORANA KUKA EPSTEIN, MD
Director, Hair Center Serbia, Belgrade, Serbia;
Director, Department of Research, Foundation
for Hair Restoration, Miami, Florida, USA;
Director, Department of Research, Foundation
for Hair Restoration, New York, New York, USA

JEFFREY S. EPSTEIN, MD
Assistant Clinical Professor, Department of
Otolaryngology, University of Miami, Miami,
Florida, USA; Director, Foundation for Hair
Restoration, Miami, Florida, USA; Director,
Foundation for Hair Restoration, New York,
New York, USA

C. WILLIAM HANKE, MD, MPH, FACP
Laser and Skin Center of Indiana, Carmel, Indiana, USA; Director, ACGME Micrographic Surgery, Dermatologic Oncology Fellowship Training Program, St. Vincent Hospital, Indianapolis, Indiana, USA; Visiting Professor of Dermatology, University of Iowa Carver College of Medicine, Iowa City, Iowa, USA; Visiting Professor of Dermatology, University of Cincinnati College of Medicine, Cincinnati, Ohio, USA

GREGORY S. KELLER, MD, FACS
Clinical Professor and Co-Director of the Facial Plastic Surgery Fellowship, Department of Head and Neck Surgery, Division of Facial Plastic Surgery, David Geffen School of Medicine, University of California, Los Angeles, Los Angeles, USA; Attending Physician, Cottage Hospital, Santa Barbara, Santa Barbara, California, USA

SAJJAD KHAN, MD
Medcare Hospital, Dubai, United Arab Emirates

MATT LEAVITT, DO
Founder, CEO, Advanced Dermatology and Cosmetic Surgery, Executive Medical Advisor, Bosley, Maitland, Florida, USA; KCU-GME/ADCS Orlando Dermatology Residency, Associate Clinical Professor, University of Central Florida, Nova Southeastern University, Orlando, Florida, USA

JIAHUI LIN, MD
Resident, Department of Otolaryngology–Head and Neck Surgery, Weill Cornell Medicine, New York, New York, USA

VISHAD NABILI, MD
Professor, Division of Facial Plastic and Reconstructive Surgery, Department of Head and Neck Surgery, David Geffen School of Medicine, University of California, Los Angeles, Los Angeles, California, USA

ANDREA M. PARK, MD
Division of Facial Plastic Surgery, Department of Otolaryngology–Head and Neck Surgery, David Geffen School of Medicine, University of California, Los Angeles, Los Angeles, California, USA

KIM PHAM, MPH
University of Wisconsin-Madison, School of Medicine and Public Health, Madison, Wisconsin, USA

JOHN D. RACHEL, MD
Facial Plastics, Chicago, Illinois, USA

JEFFREY RAWNSLEY, MD
Department of Otolaryngology–Head and Neck Surgery, Division of Facial Plastic and Reconstructive Surgery, University of California, Los Angeles, Los Angeles, California, USA

MICHAEL SACOPULOS, JD
President, Medical Risk Management, Medical Risk Institute, Terre Haute, Indiana, USA

JORDAN P. SAND, MD
Spokane Center for Facial Plastic Surgery, Spokane, Washington, USA; Department of Otolaryngology–Head and Neck Surgery, University of Washington School of Medicine, Seattle, Washington, USA

ANTHONY P. SCLAFANI, MD
Professor and Director of Facial Plastic Surgery, Department of Otolaryngology–Head and Neck Surgery, Weill Cornell Medicine, New York, New York, USA

AMY FORMAN TAUB, MD
Assistant Clinical Professor, Department of Dermatology, Northwestern University Feinberg School of Medicine, Chicago, Illinois, USA; Founder/Director, Advanced Dermatology, Lincolnshire, Illinois, USA; Founder/Director, Advanced Dermatology, Glencoe, Illinois, USA

JILL WAIBEL, MD
Medical Director, Dermatology, Miami Dermatology and Laser Institute, Subsection Chief of Dermatology, Baptist Hospital of Miami, Assistant Professor, Miller School of Medicine, University of Miami, Miami, Florida, USA

DAVID A. WOLF, MD, EE
NASA/White House Advisor on Space Policy, Former Astronaut and Chief of NASA Stem Cell Research, Johnson Space Center, Astronaut, President and CEO, EarthTomorrow, Inc, Houston, Texas, USA; Visiting Professor, Purdue University, West Lafayette, Indiana, USA

Contents

from the lipoaspirate. The regenerative, antiinflammatory, and immunomodulatory effects of the stromal vascular fraction are being documented in ongoing therapeutic response studies.

The current state of the applicability of cell therapy for the treatment of various conditions of hair loss reveals a promising and potentially effective role. Further research, based on published work to date, is indicated to explore the potential roles of autologous fat grafting, mesenchymal stem cells, and stromal vascular fraction therapy. The authors' evolving experience matches these promising scientific findings.

The use of stem cells in regenerative medicine and specifically facial rejuvenation is thought provoking and controversial. There is increased emphasis on tissue engineering and regenerative medicine, which translates into a need for a reliable source of stem cells in addition to biomaterial scaffolds and cytokine growth factors. Adipose tissue is currently recognized as an accessible and abundant source for adult stem cells. Cellular therapies and tissue engineering are still in their infancy, and additional basic science and preclinical studies are needed before cosmetic and reconstructive surgical applications can be routinely undertaken and satisfactory levels of patient safety achieved.

FACIAL PLASTIC SURGERY CLINICS OF NORTH AMERICA

SERIES OF RELATED INTEREST

Clinics in Plastic Surgery
Available at: https://www.plasticsurgery.theclinics.com/
Otolaryngologic Clinics
Available at: https://www.oto.theclinics.com/

THE CLINICS ARE AVAILABLE ONLINE!
Access your subscription at:
www.theclinics.com

Preface
Biologic Treatments Are Our Future, but a More Regulated One

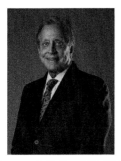

Gregory S. Keller, MD, FACS
Editor

There is very little question that development of biological products is a large part of facial plastic surgery's future. Our colleagues in plastic surgery have embraced these technologies and are moving forward with them.

The younger members of physicians practicing facial plastic surgery will see a remarkable advance in biological reconstruction and manipulation of tissue beyond the practice of fat transplantation. In fact, clinical uses of biologicals (other than fat) are now entering the "mainstream." Even tissue engineering, such as manufacturing autologous grafts for severely burned patients (Epicell; Genzyme Biosurgery, Cambridge, MA, USA), is currently available to the clinician. It may be that the twentieth century was the "age of transplantation" and the twenty-first will be the age of autologous synthetic reconstruction of organs, cartilage, skin, and the like.

The use of platelet-rich plasma, stromal vascular fraction, fat, growth factors, peptides, and mesothelial stem cells is now quite common. This issue of *Facial Plastic Surgery Clinics of North America* is an attempt to introduce current uses of biologicals, and to interest and inform facial plastic surgeons about the biologic basis and clinical use of these products. Another hope is to inspire younger surgeons to pursue biologics.

My interest in biologicals began in the early 1990s. It was at the December 1994 second meeting of a new organization (A4M), that I was asked to speak on endoscopic surgery by Vince Giampappa, MD, a plastic surgeon who was on the program committee. After interfacing with several PhDs, who were pioneers in embryonic stem cell work and telomerase, I became intently interested in finding clinical applications for biologicals and cellular products.

After interaction and collaboration with a Russian scientist at UCLA, we began work with fibroblasts and liver cells. The challenges of working with product development, and the reality of bringing biologicals to clinical usage and acceptance, evolved over this time. These challenges have changed and evolved, but these same challenges persist to this day. For a biological to reach clinical usage, it must overcome the following hurdles:

1. Basic Science Safety and Efficacy: For biologicals to be effective, they must provide a potential clinical benefit. Our current scientific knowledge base needs to not only support the premise of clinical benefit but also demonstrate that the product does not produce clinical harm. This is especially important in the elective and aesthetic areas of practice.
2. Development: Manufacturing of the product is as difficult as the science. A way to produce a clean and reproducible product with consistent, stable qualities is always a challenge for the engineers, biochemists, and pharmacologists.

Facial Plast Surg Clin N Am 26 (2018) ix–xi
https://doi.org/10.1016/j.fsc.2018.06.012
1064-7406/18/© 2018 Published by Elsevier Inc.

3. Regulatory Hurdles: Formerly, autologous products did not require US Food and Drug Administration (FDA) regulation. Initially, autologous fibroblasts, chondrocytes, and skin cells for burn victims were available to the clinical market. Biopsies were taken, and the target cells were expanded in culture (some added to matrices) and reimplanted. After these products' introduction and marketing, a new division of the FDA was formed to regulate "biologicals," and these products were removed from the market and subjected to similar regulatory status as drugs. Autologous tissues removed from the patient and reimplanted at the same surgical event (such as fat transplantation) were, however, allowed. Transplantation of hearts, kidneys, bone marrow, blood transfusions and banking, fat, and so forth did not require regulation different from that already in place. Recently, with the evolution of biologicals (and clinical experience in other countries of potential adverse effects) the FDA has increased its regulation of both the biologicals and the medical devices used in production and implantation of biologicals. One can only expect regulation of biologicals to increase, possibly improving safety, but also delaying development of new technologies. Many American physicians (me included) have avoided potential FDA conflicts by ceasing to advance product development, and it is possible that the "cutting edge" of technologies will be shifted to other countries. Cooperation and partnership with the FDA is an integral part of clinical development in this day and age.

4. Ethics and Religion: The ethics of development in the past were largely left to the physician and his adherence to the Hippocratic Oath, which every medical student took upon matriculation from medical school Subsequently, IRB's and ethical panels were developed to reflect not only medical ethics but also community ethics and values as well. These ethics and values often change over time, but are of great benefit in bringing medical technology into community acceptance. A potential negative aspect of this is the ongoing deprecation of industry, which as noted above, is a source of medical development. Lack of industry participation, especially with the current decrease in government funding, can stall clinical applications with the lack of developmental funds for projects that are not extremely profitable. Similar barriers to medical development occur with the religious and political opinions of the United States and other countries that impede the use of biologicals, particularly stem cells. Despite the fact that it is no longer necessary to utilize fertilized stem cells, many religious groups feel that multipotent stem cells should not reach clinical usage. Today, it is imperative to weigh the medical, religious, ethical, and community values and form acceptable partnerships with these entities.

5. Clinical Acceptance: Clinical acceptance usually means a series of studies that demonstrate safety and efficacy. Since the early 1900s, the medical community has appropriately demanded scientific evidence. As mentioned above, the barriers to biological development discussed above make studies more difficult to complete, as the complexity and cost of bringing a product to clinical usage increases.

6. Industry Acceptance and Marketing (ie, Profitability): Unless a product is profitable, it will not reach the market or last long in the marketplace. Autologous fibroblasts for acne scars and wrinkle fill are a case in point. After years of FDA trials and clinical studies, the amortized costs of research and development, the need for biopsy, and cell growth under stringent manufacturing conditions, the cost of biopsy and tissue expansion in the laboratory facility and the subsequent implantation, injections require a price point that is often too expensive to justify routine use (Laviv; Fibrocell Technologies, Exton, PA, USA). When the product went to market in the 1990s, prior to the above barriers, it was profitable to spend the money marketing it at a reasonable price point. After the barriers were instituted, it was not able to sustain a marketable price point for routine use; all of this, despite the fact that it was a treatment that has yet to be duplicated in long-term efficacy. I personally retain fibroblast fill in my scars and nasolabial folds over 20 years later. Another problem for industry is that the cost to market any product has increased. Industry must now go "direct to consumer" with Internet, television, and print advertising, in addition to the former scientific presentations. This narrows the number of "orphan" biologicals that industry can sustain.

The "good" of all of this is that the American consumer is clearly protected to a greater degree than previously. The "bad" is that it is much more difficult and expensive to bring a product to market.

Despite all of these problems, many biological products are now generally accepted into clinical usage. In this issue, our purpose is to cover some of the basic science of hair and skin and to cover clinical applications that are currently in use, and, of which many plastic surgeons may not be aware. It is also to encourage facial plastic surgeons to evolve usage of these products, as they are, without a doubt in my mind, our future.

Update Addendum: This preface turned out to be somewhat prophetic. Since the date of this submission, the FDA has clearly moved to further regulate the production and usage of stem cells for certain treatments that, in the FDA's mind, are "unproven." In May, the FDA filed injunctions on two nationwide chains of clinics that are based in Florida and California (https://www.cnn.com/2018/05/10/health/fda-complaints-stem-cell-clinics/index.html). The agency has issued previous warnings about the unproven uses of stem cells. A well-publicized case of blindness following an injection of fat-derived stromal vascular fraction (mesothelial stem cells, fibroblasts, and other cells) may have precipitated the FDA's actions (https://www.theatlantic.com/science/archive/2017/10/stem-cell-eye/541299/). While injections of platelet-rich plasma, nonmodified fat, nonmodified autologous tissue, such as cartilage, and localized mesothelial stem cell injections for localized orthopedic problems have escaped scrutiny, it appears that the FDA is involved in deriving new regulations to regulate biologic tissues that are designed to protect consumers. As physicians in the twenty-first century, we are required to "first do no harm" and update our research protocols to match the current levels of scrutiny.

Gregory S. Keller, MD, FACS
Keller Facial Plastic Surgery
221 West Pueblo Street
Santa Barbara, CA 93105, USA

E-mail address:
gsk@gregorykeller.com

Introduction: An Overview

Gregory S. Keller, MD*, Andrea M. Park, MD

KEYWORDS

- Biologics • Overview • Clinical use • Biologicals

KEY POINTS

- Clinical use of biologicals is rapidly increasing.
- The earliest approaches to facial rejuvenation involved invoking the responses of wound healing and repair.
- Biologicals act by directly depositing growth factors, peptides, and stem cells into a given area, often without inflammation and repair.

The use of biologicals for clinical use is rapidly increasing. One of the logical questions is what constitutes a biological? The official definition of biological products by the Food and Drug Administration (FDA) is "Biological products can be composed of sugars, proteins, or nucleic acids, or a combination of these substances. They may also be living entities, such as cells and tissues. Biologics are made from a variety of natural resources—human, animal, and microorganism may be produced by biotechnology methods."

Within this rather all-encompassing definition, there is a subset of biological products that are in clinical use in facial plastic surgery. These products are primarily peptides, cytokines, growth factors, interleukins, proteins, and cells. Proteins are larger chains of amino acids that are not easily transported through the skin. In skin, proteins form and regulate the extracellular matrix, the basement membrane of the skin, and the adhesions of cell-to-cell relations.

Peptides are smaller chains of amino acids that include cytokines and growth factors. Cytokines are secreted glycoproteins that are produced by a broad range of cells, including immune cells like macrophages, B lymphocytes, T lymphocytes, and mast cells as well as endothelial cells, fibroblasts, and various stromal cells. They are often first responders in signaling the inflammation pathway and regulate it.

A growth factor is a naturally occurring protein capable of stimulating and regulating cellular growth, proliferation, healing, and cellular differentiation. Growth factors typically act as signaling molecules between cells and have receptors that bind them. Growth factors are often released by activated platelets. An individual growth factor may stimulate multiple cellular reactions. Peptides are usually smaller chains of amino acids that have relatively more narrow signaling capabilities on tissue. Antimicrobial peptides, such as defensins, have effects on singular reparative processes that may proceed without inflammation.

The skin is a complex structure of cells supported in an extracellular matrix (ECM) that provides a scaffold of support and an organizational matrix for the skin organ. Fibroblasts produce the matrix proteins that make up much of the ECM.

Stem cells are cells that are responsible for generating tissues and are generally classified as pluripotent (embryonic stem cells, induced stem cells, cloned stem cells, umbilical stem cells, and so forth), multipotent, or unipotent. An embryonic (or pluripotent) stem cell can evolve into a tree option of differentiation, initially

Disclosure Statement: Dr G.S. Keller acknowledges a conflict of interest in being a founder and possessing an ownership interest in Medicell Technologies, producer of DefenAge.

Division of Facial Plastic Surgery, Department of Head and Neck Surgery, David Geffen School of Medicine, University of California, Los Angeles, Los Angeles, CA, USA

* Corresponding author. 221 West Pueblo Street, Suite A, Santa Barbara, CA 93105.

E-mail address: faclft@aol.com

Facial Plast Surg Clin N Am 26 (2018) 403–405
https://doi.org/10.1016/j.fsc.2018.06.001

branching into an ectodermal, mesodermal, or endodermal pathway. From this, further differentiation to a specific structure develops via a complex series of differentiations along the tree. Progenitor cells are cells along the differentiation pathway and can be cultured and multiplied to travel to a more limited pathway than the pluripotent stem cell (**Fig. 1**).

Adult stem cells are cells that are present in adult tissues. These cells, such as the basal cell in skin, are responsible for maintaining and regenerating the skin and underlying structures. These stem cells may also age but are targets for numerous biological treatments. Other skin stem cells within the skin and subcutaneous tissue are held in reserve for crises, such as injuries and infections, and are not as susceptible to the aging processes.

The skin is composed of dermis, epidermis, and subcutaneous tissue. The epidermis is the protective layer of the skin that provides a barrier to harmful effects, such as an infectious agent, water loss, dryness, and so forth. The basal layer of the skin is the bottom layer of the 5 layers of the epidermis, and basal cells are adult stem cells that produce keratinocytes. These cells evolve into cells of the spinous, granular, and horny layers, in the continual evolution and turnover of the skin.

The principal cell in the dermis is the fibroblast; it produces most of the proteins of the dermis, such as collagens and elastins, and enzymes, such as collagenases. In the papillary dermis, fibroblasts are varied; but in the reticular dermis, fibroblasts have more myofibroblast characteristics for contraction and scarring. Immune cells, such as neutrophils, macrophages, and the like, are also present here. With aging, fibroblasts senesce and the dermal ECM diminishes. The dermis loses its thickness, and the skin appears thinner and wrinkles appear.

In the subcutaneous tissue, fat, sweat glands, and hair follicles are present. These structures are repositories of stem cells, fat cells, and collagen. This layer, with aging, diminishes in thickness, with an apparent loss of volume to the facial features. With aging, hair follicles miniaturize and hairs grow shorter, thinner, fall out entirely, and lose pigmentation.

The earliest approaches to facial rejuvenation involved invoking the responses of wound healing and repair. Wound healing undergoes a progression of hemostasis, inflammation, proliferation, and remodeling with a complex interaction of growth factors, peptides, cellular response, and migration.

Chemical peeling is one of the first forms of rejuvenation that used the mechanism of inflammation and repair. Cleopatra was rumored to use lactic acid peels to smooth her skin, and various types of chemicals were used in the nineteenth century in Europe.

Chemical peeling causes skin damage using caustic agents. Also called chemexfoliation, skin damage is caused by caustic agents in a more or less semicontrolled fashion.

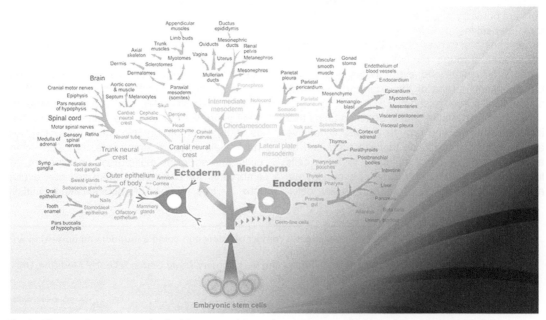

Fig. 1. Bio-tree. Symp, sympathetic. (*Courtesy of* Ascendance Bio, Inc, Alameda, CA; with permission.)

The resulting process of inflammation and repair results in the induction of a cellular response resulting in the release of cytokines. The subsequent cascade of cellular processes stimulates an ultimate thickening of the dermis and epidermis, collagen deposition, and structural reorganization.

Heat and injury, induced by lasers, radiofrequency, and microwave devices, also cause the cascade of events that results in inflammation and repair. These effects modify (each device in a different, defined, and engineered manner) the collagen, elastin, and ECM of the skin. With the process of inflammation and repair, growth factors, peptides, and other cellular elements stimulate rejuvenation and modification of the skin.

Biologicals act by directly depositing growth factors, peptides, and stem cells into a given area, often without inflammation and repair. Many directly encourage adult stem cells and mesothelial stem cells to initiate rejuvenation of the skin.

The current uses of biologicals mainly involve the use of platelet-rich plasma, peptides, growth factors, and mesothelial stem cells to improve skin quality, wound healing, and hair growth. These mesothelial stem cells were originally obtained from bone marrow but are currently obtained from fat tissue, for the most part. Mesothelial stem cells are multipotent and can differentiate (often combined with epidermal growth factor) into multiple cells and tissues, including adipose cells (fat), chondrocytes (cartilage), osteoblasts (bone), and muscle.

Stromal vascular fraction is a multicell product derived from processing fat. It contains adipose-derived mesothelial stem cells, endothelial progenitor cells, T cells, β cells, mast cells, and macrophages. It is currently used primarily in orthopedics but has had initial forays into plastic and aesthetic surgery uses as well. Burns, lipo-augmentation, and wound healing are 3 current target areas for mesothelial stem cell use.

Peptides, growth factors, and cosmeceuticals are also in widespread clinical use for wound healing, hair growth, and skin rejuvenation.

This issue explores the clinical use of biologics for clinical treatment. Not all of these uses are approved by the FDA and can be off label or under investigation. Some are in the cosmeceutical or hair growth realm and do not require approval, only demonstrations of safety and documentable claims that can be accepted by the FDA as aesthetic and not used for the treatment of disease.

A few of the articles in this issue are not mainstream but are included, as they have the potential to make the clinician (particularly the younger clinician) aware of treatments that are occurring and the science that is driving them.

Regretfully missing in this issue is an article on biosynthesis of cartilage, skin, hair, and bone. The original intent of this issue was to cover newer technologies that were already in clinical practice, particularly in the realm of skin and facial aging.

How to Use Oral and Topical Cosmeceuticals to Prevent and Treat Skin Aging

Leslie Baumann, MD

KEYWORDS

- Skin care • Cosmeceutical • Baumann Skin Type • Antiaging • Photoaging • Supplement
- Skin care • Improve outcome

KEY POINTS

- Keratinocytes and fibroblasts play a role in skin aging.
- DNA damage, free radicals, inflammation, and glycation cause skin aging.
- Genes, growth factors, cytokines, and stem cells (LGR6+) play a role in skin aging.
- Diet, supplements, and topical cosmeceuticals can help prevent and treat skin aging.
- Patient education and compliance are critical to improve outcomes and prevent skin aging.

INTRODUCTION

Patients should adopt strategies to decrease their risk of skin aging in their early 30s, if not sooner. It is important to identify patients at an increased risk of skin aging early enough to initiate countermeasures. The Baumann Skin Type Indicator questionnaire can be used to identify patients who are a wrinkle-prone Baumann Skin Type,[1] which is defined as more than 30 years of age and/or younger than 30 years of age with lifestyle factors putting them at an increased risk for skin aging.[2] Consistent daily use of efficacious technologies targeted to patients' Baumann Skin Type can prevent and treat many of the signs of skin aging. Patient education is also critical for success because compliance with treatment regimens is notoriously low among patients.[3]

There are several causes of skin aging that can be broken down into 2 broad categories, intrinsic and extrinsic. *Intrinsic aging* results from cellular processes that occur over time and is influenced by genetics and includes decreased function of keratinocytes and fibroblasts, intracellular and extracellular accumulation of by-products, decreased function of sirtuins, mitochondrial damage, and loss of telomeres.

Extrinsic aging is incurred through environmental causes of cell damage, including ultraviolet (UV) light and infrared and radiation exposure. Air pollution, smoking, tanning beds, sun exposure, alcohol and drugs, stress, and poor diet play a role. Extrinsic aging occurs from the interplay of overlapping processes caused by free radicals, DNA damage, glycation, inflammation, and other actions by the immune system. In most cases, these factors can be lessened through behavioral change. As much as 80% of facial aging is thought to be attributable to sun exposure.[4] Several mechanisms by which sun exposure causes aging are well understood. DNA damage results when UV light induces covalent bonds between nucleic acid base pairs and forms thymine dimers, which can alter the function of the tumor suppressor gene p53 increasing the risk of skin cancer and skin aging.[5] UV exposure also produces free

Disclosure Statement: Patent owner of patent number US 20160128925 A1 Optimized Skincare Regimens for Changing the Genetic Skin Type to the Ideal Skin Type–Oily, Resistant, Non-Pigmented and Tight Skin.
Division of Cosmetic Dermatology, University of Miami, 4500 Biscayne Boulevard Suite 101, Miami, FL 33137, USA
E-mail address: DrB@Derm.Net

Facial Plast Surg Clin N Am 26 (2018) 407–413
https://doi.org/10.1016/j.fsc.2018.06.002

radicals that cause damaging oxidative stress[6] that can lead to activation of the arachidonic acid pathway resulting in inflammation.[7] Other mechanisms of skin aging are not as well understood. This article discusses the mechanisms that play a role in aging and describes cosmeceutical interventions that have been developed to target both intrinsic and extrinsic aging. The deleterious effects of sun exposure and the need for consistent sun protective behavior including sunscreen are extremely important but are not discussed in detail in this article.

CELLS IN SKIN AGING
Keratinocytes

The epidermis is composed of keratinocyte cells found in layers that resemble the brick-and-mortar structure of a brick wall. Each epidermal layer has specific characteristics. The top layer of the epidermis, known as the stratum corneum, is particularly important because it forms the skin barrier. This protective barrier has cross-linked proteins for strength, antioxidants to protect the cells from free radicals, a bilayer lipid membrane layer to prevent water evaporation from the cellular surface, immune cells, antimicrobial peptides, and a natural microbiome. Damage to any layer of the epidermis has repercussions that can lead to increased skin aging.

Fibroblasts

The dermis is made up of fibroblast cells. These cells are like factories because they produce collagen, elastin, hyaluronic acid, heparan sulfate, and other glycosaminoglycans that keep the skin smooth, strong, and healthy. Collagen provides strength, elastin provides elasticity, and the glycosaminoglycans like hyaluronic acid, heparan sulfate (HS), and dermatan sulfate bind water, impart volume to the skin, and provide support for important cell-to-cell communication.

When keratinocytes and fibroblasts age, they get lazy and stop listening to cellular signals, such as growth factors. The main goal of any anti-aging skin care regimen is to protect and rejuvenate these important skin cells.

Cellular Damage That Leads to Aging

Accumulated damage due to intrinsic or extrinsic factors results in keratinocytes and fibroblasts that fail to produce important cellular components as well as they did when they were younger. The cellular issues that lead to aging cells are nuclear DNA damage, mitochondrial DNA damage, decreased lysosomal function, structural damage

to proteins, and damage to cell membranes. This damage occurs because of the direct effects of UV radiation, pollution, toxins, free radicals (oxidation), glycation, and inflammation.

ADDRESSING SPECIFIC CAUSES OF AGING WITH ORAL AND TOPICAL AGENTS
Preventing and Treating DNA Damage

DNA damage manifests as thymine-thymine dimers, pyrimidine-pyrimidine dimers, damage to telomeres, or other mutations. Broad-spectrum sunscreens and sun avoidance are key in preventing DNA damage induced from exposure to UV radiation. Other cosmeceutical agents have been developed to block the effects of UV radiation or to help encourage DNA repair. Besides sunscreen, the key members of the dermatologic armamentarium against DNA damage are various antioxidants. There is a plethora of data on the protective effects of antioxidants, such as polypodium leucotomos,[8] ascorbic acid, and green tea. Other antioxidants have less data but hypothetically should have similar benefits.

Polypodium leucotomos (PL), an oral extract from ferns, has been shown to exhibit photoprotective effects at an oral dose of 7.5 mg. PL has consistently demonstrated antitumor and skin protective effects.[8] A 2004 study in humans demonstrated that 2 oral doses of PL led to a significant decrease in DNA damage after UV exposure,[9] whereas a 2017 study showed PL to protect skin DNA from UVB.[10] Although PL has shown benefits topically, it is the oral form that is most often used for skin protection.

Ascorbic acid, also known as vitamin C, has been shown to provide benefits when given both orally and topically. It requires an acidic environment for optimal absorption. Topical application of ascorbic acid, vitamin E, and ferulic acid has been shown to decrease the formation of thymine dimers.[11] Ascorbic acid is unique when compared with other antioxidants because it also stimulates procollagen genes in fibroblasts prodding them to increase collagen synthesis.[12]

Niacinamide, also known as nicotinamide, is an important part of the niacin coenzymes nicotinamide adenine dinucleotide (NAD+), NAD+ phosphate (NADP+), and their reduced forms NADH and NADPH. These coenzymes play a role in DNA synthesis and repair in addition to being involved in hundreds of other important enzymatic reactions. Topical niacinamide has been shown to play a role in DNA repair[13] by giving the cells the energy that the DNA repair enzymes need to unwind the DNA strand, replace the nucleosides, and rewind the strand. Specifically, niacinamide has been shown to increase DNA excision repair and enhance repair of cyclobutane pyrimidine dimers (caused by UVB) and 8-oxo-7,8-dihydro-2′-deoxyguanosine (caused by UVA).[14] Niacinamide is used topically because oral forms of niacin are associated with flushing.

Green tea has an active component known as EpiGalloCatechin-3-O-Gallate, which has been shown to induce interleukin 12 to increase the production of enzymes that repair UV-induced DNA damage.[15] The proven photoprotective effects of topical and oral green tea include reduction of UV-induced erythema, diminished sunburn cell formation, and a decrease in DNA damage.[16]

Preventing and Treating Mitochondrial DNA Damage

UV radiation causes mitochondrial DNA damage known as an mtDNA common deletion.[17] Mitochondria with the common deletion produce damaging free radicals known as reactive oxygen species (ROS). Mitochondria damage due to ROS decreases the mitochondria's ability to generate energy in the form of ATP. ATP is the form of energy required for DNA repair and other reparative processes.

Free radicals and UV radiation are the primary cause of harm to the mitochondria. Normal cellular metabolism results in harm to the mitochondria. The cascade of damage includes mitochondrial DNA impairment, loss of mitochondrial enzymes, and reduced ATP production. This damage results in less energy for DNA repair and corresponding cellular lethargy. Unfortunately, there is no proven way to reduce mitochondrial damage once it has occurred, although many research initiatives to do exactly this are underway. At this point, protecting the mitochondria from harm with sunscreens and antioxidants is critical.

Antioxidants should be used to thwart the effects of free radicals on vulnerable mitochondria. Coenzyme Q_{10} (CoQ_{10}) is particularly useful because it is a component of the mitochondrial respiratory chain in addition to being an antioxidant. CoQ_{10} is found in both oral and topical formulations. If taken orally, it should only be used in the morning because of a caffeine-type effect. Topical forms of CoQ_{10} have a dark yellow color that may make them less appealing to patients. PL has been shown to decrease the amount of common deletions found in the mitochondria of irradiated keratinocytes and fibroblasts.[18] The oral form should be used. Curcumin is being investigated for mitochondrial protective effects.[19] Its strong yellow color and smell make it more suited for oral use, although many companies are trying to develop cosmetically elegant topical formulations.

Scavenging Free Radicals

UV light, pollution, and other insults cause formation of free radicals. Even sunscreen use has been associated with increased formation of free radicals. Free radicals, also known as ROS, cause damage to cells in many ways, including mitochondrial damage, DNA mutations, glycation, lysosomal damage, and oxidation of important lipids and other cellular components, such as proteins. Antioxidants have a multitude of beneficial effects, including scavenging free radicals, decreasing activation of mitogen-activated protein kinases, chelation of copper required by tyrosinase, and suppression of inflammatory factors, such as nuclear factor (NF)-κB.[20] Antioxidants are critical in the prevention of aged skin.

Preventing and Treating Inflammation

Inflammation leads to skin aging via several mechanisms, including formation of ROS. There are multiple etiologic pathways that lead to inflammation. The process is orchestrated by a large array of inflammatory mediators, including histamines, cytokines, eicosanoids (eg, prostaglandins, thromboxanes, and leukotrienes), complement cascade components, kinins, fibrinopeptide enzymes, NF-κB, and free radicals. The various inflammatory cascades participate in a domino effect resulting in a convoluted inflammatory process. One example is the cascade that is triggered by UV light and free radicals when they oxidize cell membrane lipids leading to the release of arachidonic acid. The arachidonic acid cascade plays an important role in skin inflammation because it activates cyclooxygenase-2 (COX-2) resulting in production of inflammation-causing compounds, such as prostaglandins and leukotrienes, that recruit inflammatory immune cells to the area. NF-κB is another key regulator of inflammation in the skin.[20]

Antiinflammatory ingredients used successfully in topical skin care include argan oil, caffeine, chamomile, feverfew, green tea, licorice extract, aloe, linoleic acid (found in high concentrations in argan oil and safflower oil), and niacinamide. Oral PL has been shown to block the effect of UV radiation on the expression of COX-2.[21] Glycolic acid has been shown to suppress COX-2 signaling and other inflammatory mediators.[22]

Preventing and Treating Glycation

Glycation is caused by the Maillard reaction, a chemical reaction between an amino acid and a sugar that usually requires heat and is a well-known phenomenon in cooking. Louis-Camille Maillard first described this reaction in 1912 when he observed that amino acids can react with sugar to create brown or golden-brown compounds. Scientists recognized the importance of glycation in health in the 1980s.

When glycation occurs, sugar molecules attach to proteins, thus initiating a series of chemical reactions. These cross-linked proteins are called advanced glycation end products. This occurs in collagen fibers and results in the formation of cross-links that bind collagen fibers to each other, in turn, rendering the skin stiffer. Glycosylated collagen is thought to play a role in the appearance of aged skin.[23] Elastin can also be affected by glycation. Photoaged skin has an impaired ability to rebound and when seen under a microscope exhibits elastin that is abnormally clumped together. This condition is known as elastosis. Recent research has found that these clumps are likely caused by glycation, because the adhering elastin is stiff and devoid of its usual springiness, which is likely the reason that diabetes is associated with increased skin aging compared with normal controls. Therefore, glycation most likely plays a role in the damage seen in the collagen and elastin of aged skin.

Many antiaging skin care products claim to treat glycation, but unfortunately it is not a reversible reaction. Prevention is key. Some studies suggest that antioxidants may play a role; however, it is more likely that they just divert the process down a different pathway that ultimately culminates in glycation anyway. Lowering serum glucose levels is the best way to prevent glycation.[24] Dietary intervention and oral metformin have been recommended to decrease glycation.

REVERSING THE EFFECTS OF AGING ON SKIN CELLS
Role of Epidermal Keratinocytes in Aging

Young basal stem cells produce many new keratinocytes resulting in fast cell turnover and robust production of protective epidermal components. Old keratinocytes exhibit less energy, become less responsive to cellular signals, and do not produce important protective components.[25,26] Keratinocyte stem cell function is diminished with age and damage that accumulates over time, characterized by a decreased response to growth factors, reduced keratinization, and impaired function.[27]

Role of Dermal Fibroblasts in Skin Aging

Young fibroblasts synthesize important cellular components, including collagen, elastin, hyaluronic acid, and heparan sulfate. Production decreases in older fibroblasts. Like aged keratinocytes, old fibroblasts lose energy and become less responsive to growth factors and other cellular signals.[25,26]

Rejuvenating Aged Skin with Cosmeceuticals

Gene expression, growth factors, cytokines, chemokines, and receptor activation direct the function of keratinocytes and fibroblasts. To reverse or slow cellular skin aging, these old keratinocytes and fibroblasts need to be stimulated to respond to these signals or the signals need to be increased.

Stimulating old keratinocytes and fibroblasts
The necessary conditions for stimulating aged keratinocytes and fibroblasts include activating gene expression, adding growth factors, activating cytokines and chemokines, turning on receptors, and making cells more responsive to signals.

Influencing gene expression
Retinoids have been shown to influence collagen genes and increase activity of procollagen genes and decrease production of collagenase. Many studies have demonstrated the efficacy of retinoids to treat aged skin[13] and to prevent skin aging. This has been shown in both sun-exposed and non–sun-exposed areas.[28] Both prescription retinoids (tretinoin, adapalene, tazarotene) and over-the-counter retinoids (retinol) should be the first choice to treat and prevent aging by stimulating old keratinocytes and fibroblasts.[28,29] However, stimulating the retinoic acid receptors with retinoids will almost invariably lead to redness and flaking in the first few weeks. For this reason, retinoids should be titrated slowly. Retinoid esters, such as retinyl palmitate and retinyl linoleate, do not penetrate into the dermis[30] and are not as effective as retinol, tretinoin, adapalene, and tazarotene. Retinol is available without a prescription and is less costly than the prescribed forms of retinoids; therefore, retinol use likely results in increased compliance as compared with other forms of topical retinoids.

Alpha hydroxy acids are also capable of stimulating collagen genes to increase collagen production.[31–33] In addition, ascorbic acid has been shown to stimulate collagen genes resulting in increased type 1 collagen production by fibroblasts.[34]

Growth factors

Using cosmetic products that contain growth factors can also achieve skin rejuvenation. There are many types of growth factors to stimulate old keratinocytes and fibroblasts to increase function.[35] Growth factors may directly stimulate genes or may act as a signaling mechanism. Growth factors are inactive or susceptible to degradation in their native, soluble form. To exert their quintessential functions, they must be presented to the correct receptor site in order for the cell to hear their signal.[36]

Heparan sulfate

HS has an important role in cell-to-cell communications. It increases the cellular response to growth factors[36] by helping the old, lazy fibroblasts hear the cellular signals better. HS binds, stores, and protects growth factors, allowing them to complete transport to their targets, and then presents them to the proper binding site.[36,37] A topically applied analogue of HS has been shown to rejuvenate aged skin.[38]

Stem cells

Stem cells contained in cosmeceutical products are typically derived from plants, are too large to penetrate the stratum corneum, have short shelf lives, and do not function as human stem cells would. For this reason, stem cells in cosmeceuticals are virtually useless. However, new technologies have revealed ingredients that can stimulate the native stem cells to repopulate the epidermis and dermis with young cells. Skin stem cells in skin include basal stem cells and 10 types of hair follicle stem cells. The LGR6+ hair follicle cells play an important role in repopulating the epidermis after wounding.[39,40] For years aesthetic physicians have known that wounding the skin with lasers, needles, and acidic peels will improve its appearance. New data have shown that wounding the skin stimulates LGR6+ stem cells to repopulate the epidermis. When wounding occurs, neutrophils release a peptide known as defensin. Defensin stimulates the LGR6+ stem cells to repopulate the epidermis.[41] Topical defensin, formulated in a preparation to allow penetration into hair follicles where the LGR6+ stem cells reside, has been shown to give the skin a smoother, more youthful appearance.

SUMMARY

Identifying patients at risk for skin aging early is important. Getting them started on a consistent and correct skin care regimen consisting of a daily sunscreen of 15 or higher, a nightly topical retinoid, and oral and topical antioxidants are the minimum requirements. Combining these with cleansers, moisturizers, and treatment products with hydroxy acids, growth factors, heparan sulfate, and defensin should be done according to the patients' other skin type parameters, such as dryness, inflammation, and melanocyte activity. Multiple studies show that patients display poor compliance.[42,43] Educating them about the need for skin protection and giving them printed instructions is the key to improving compliance.[44] The ultimate goal is to promote healthy lifestyle habits and encourage compliance with scientifically proven antiaging therapies.

REFERENCES

1. Baumann L. Cosmeceuticals and cosmetic ingredients. New York: McGraw Hill Professional; 2014.
2. Baumann LS. The baumann skin typing system. In: Farage MA, Miller K, Maibach H, et al, editors. Textbook of aging skin. Berlin: Springer-Verlag; 2017. p. 1579–94.
3. Storm A, Benfeldt E, Andersen SE, et al. A prospective study of patient adherence to topical treatments: 95% of patients underdose. J Am Acad Dermatol 2008;59(6):975–80.
4. Uitto J. Understanding premature skin aging. N Engl J Med 1997;337:1463.
5. Tornaletti S, Pfeifer GP. Slow repair of pyrimidine dimers at p53 mutation hotspots in skin cancer. Science 1994;263:1436–8.
6. Bickers DR, Athar M. Oxidative stress in the pathogenesis of skin disease. J Investig Dermatol 2006; 126:2565–75.
7. Yaar M, Gilchrest BA. Photoageing, mechanism, prevention and therapy. Br J Dermatol 2007;157:874–87.
8. Parrado C, Mascaraque M, Gilaberte Y, et al. Fernblock (polypodium leucotomos Extract): molecular mechanisms and pleiotropic effects in light-related skin conditions, photoaging and skin cancers, a review. Int J Mol Sci 2016;17(7) [pii: E1026].
9. Middelkamp-Hup MA, Pathak MA, Parrado C, et al. Oral polypodium leucotomos extract decreases ultraviolet-induced damage of human skin. J Am Acad Dermatol 2004;51(6):910–8.
10. Kohli I, Shafi R, Isedeh P, et al. The impact of oral polypodium leucotomos extract on ultraviolet B response: a human clinical study. J Am Acad Dermatol 2017;77(1):33–41.
11. Murray JC, Burch JA, Streilein RD, et al. A topical antioxidant solution containing vitamins C and E stabilized by ferulic acid provides protection for human skin against damage caused by ultraviolet irradiation. J Am Acad Dermatol 2008;59(3): 418–25.
12. Geesin JC, Darr D, Kaufman R, et al. Ascorbic acid specifically increases type I and type III procollagen

messenger RNA levels in human skin fibroblast. J Invest Dermatol 1988;90(4):420–4.

13. Thompson BC, Halliday GM, Damian DL. Nicotinamide enhances repair of arsenic and ultraviolet radiation-induced DNA damage in HaCaT keratinocytes and ex vivo human skin. PLoS One 2015; 10(2):e0117491.

14. Surjana D, Halliday GM, Damian DL. Nicotinamide enhances repair of ultraviolet radiation-induced DNA damage in human keratinocytes and ex vivo skin. Carcinogenesis 2013;34(5):1144–9.

15. Meeran SM, Mantena SK, Elmets CA, et al. (-)-Epigallocatechin-3-gallate prevents photocarcinogenesis in mice through interleukin-12-dependent DNA repair. Cancer Res 2006;66(10):5512–20.

16. Elmets CA, Singh D, Tubesing K, et al. Cutaneous photoprotection from ultraviolet injury by green tea polyphenols. J Am Acad Dermatol 2001;44:425.

17. Berneburg M, Plettenberg H, Medve-König K, et al. Induction of the photoaging-associated mitochondrial common deletion in vivo in normal human skin. J Invest Dermatol 2004;122(5):1277–83.

18. Villa A, Viera MH, Amini S, et al. Decrease of ultraviolet A light-induced "common deletion" in healthy volunteers after oral Polypodium leucotomos extract supplement in a randomized clinical trial. J Am Acad Dermatol 2010;62(3):511–3.

19. Trujillo J, Granados-Castro LF, Zazueta C, et al. Mitochondria as a target in the therapeutic properties of curcumin. Arch Pharm 2014;347(12):873–84.

20. Muthusamy V, Piva TJ. The UV response of the skin, a review of the MAPK, NFκB and TNFα signal transduction pathways. Arch Dermatol Res 2010;302(1):5–17.

21. Zattra E, Coleman C, Arad S, et al. Polypodium leucotomos extract decreases UV-induced Cox-2 expression and inflammation, enhances DNA repair, and decreases mutagenesis in hairless mice. Am J Pathol 2009;175(5):1952–61.

22. Tang SC, Liao PY, Hung SJ, et al. Topical application of glycolic acid suppresses the UVB induced IL-6, IL-8, MCP-1 and COX-2 inflammation by modulating NF-κB signaling pathway in keratinocytes and mice skin. J Dermatol Sci 2017;86(3):238–48.

23. Pageon H, Bakala H, Monnier VM, et al. Collagen glycation triggers the formation of aged skin in vitro. Eur J Dermatol 2007;17:12.

24. Gkogkolou P, Böhm M. Advanced glycation end products (AGEs): emerging mediators of skin aging. In: Farage M, Miller K, Maibach H, editors. Textbook of aging skin. Berlin:Springer-Verlag; 2017. p. 1675–86.

25. Stanulis-Praeger BM, Gilchrest BA. Growth factor responsiveness declines during adulthood for human skin-derived cells. Mech Ageing Dev 1986; 35(2):185–98.

26. Reenstra WR, Yaar M, Gilchrest BA. Aging affects epidermal growth factor receptor phosphorylation and traffic kinetics. Exp Cell Res 1996;227(2):252–5.

27. Stefanato CM, Yaar M, Bhawan J, et al. Modulations of nerve growth factor and Bcl-2 in ultraviolet-irradiated human epidermis. J Cutan Pathol 2003; 30(6):351–7.

28. Kafi R, Kwak HS, Schumacher WE, et al. Improvement of naturally aged skin with vitamin A (retinol). Arch Dermatol 2007;143(5):606–12.

29. Weiss JS, Ellis CN, Headington JT, et al. Topical tretinoin improves photoaged skin. A double-blind vehicle-controlled study. JAMA 1988;259(4):527–32.

30. Duell EA, Kang S, Voorhees JJ. Unoccluded retinol penetrates human skin in vivo more effectively than unoccluded retinyl palmitate or retinoic acid. J Invest Dermatol 1997;109(3):301–5.

31. Ditre CM, Griffin TD, Murphy GF, et al. Effects of alpha-hydroxy acids on photoaged skin: a pilot clinical, histologic, and ultrastructural study. J Am Acad Dermatol 1996;34(2 Pt 1):187–95.

32. Smith WP. Epidermal and dermal effects of topical lactic acid. J Am Acad Dermatol 1996;35(3 Pt 1):388–91.

33. Bernstein EF, Lee J, Brown DB, et al. Glycolic acid treatment increases type I collagen mRNA and hyaluronic acid content of human skin. Dermatol Surg 2001;27(5):429–33.

34. Phillips CL, Combs SB, Pinnell SR. Effects of ascorbic acid on proliferation and collagen synthesis in relation to the donor age of human dermal fibroblasts. J Invest Dermatol 1994;103(2):228–32.

35. Aldag C, Nogueira Teixeira D, Leventhal PS. Skin rejuvenation using cosmetic products containing growth factors, cytokines, and matrikines: a review of the literature. Clin Cosmet Investig Dermatol 2016;9:411–9.

36. Gandhi NS, Mancera RL. The structure of glycosaminoglycans and their interactions with proteins. Chem Biol Drug Des 2008;72(6):455–82.

37. Simon Davis DA, Parish CR. Heparan sulfate: a ubiquitous glycosaminoglycan with multiple roles in immunity. Front Immunol 2013;4:470.

38. Gallo RL, Bucay VW, Shamban AT, et al. The potential role of topically applied heparan sulfate in the treatment of photodamage. J Drugs Dermatol 2015;14(7):669–74.

39. Snippert HJ, Haegebarth A, Kasper M, et al. Lgr6 marks stem cells in the hair follicle that generate all cell lineages of the skin. Science 2010; 327(5971):1385–9.

40. Lough DM, Yang M, Blum A, et al. Transplantation of the LGR6+ epithelial stem cell into full-thickness cutaneous wounds results in enhanced healing, nascent hair follicle development, and augmentation of angiogenic analytes. Plast Reconstr Surg 2014; 133(3):579–90.

41. Lough D, Dai H, Yang M, et al. Stimulation of the follicular bulge LGR5+ and LGR6+ stem cells with the gut-derived human alpha defensin 5 results in decreased bacterial presence, enhanced wound healing, and hair growth from tissues devoid of

adnexal structures. Plast Reconstr Surg 2013;
132(5):1159–71.

42. Maheshwari RK, Singh AK, Gaddipati J, et al. Multiple biological activities of curcumin: a short review.
Life Sci 2006;78:2081–7.

43. Storm A, Andersen SE, Bonfeldt E, et al. One
in 3 prescriptions are never redeemed: primary
nonadherence in an outpatient clinic. J Am Acad
Dermatol 2008;59(1):27–33.

44. Hong J, Nguyen TV, Prose NS. Compassionate
care: enhancing physician-patient communication
and education in dermatology: part II: patient
education. J Am Acad Dermatol 2013;68(3):364.
e1-10.

Hair Biology
Growth and Pigmentation

Andrea M. Park, MD[a],*, Sajjad Khan, MD[b], Jeffrey Rawnsley, MD[a]

KEYWORDS

- Hair growth cycle • Hair pigmentation • Gray hair • Hair biology • Minoxidil • Finasteride
- Dutasteride • PRP

KEY POINTS

- The 3 phases of the hair growth cycle are anagen, catagen, and telogen.
- Topical minoxidil opens potassium channels and increases the diameter of existing hairs.
- Oral finasteride is a Food and Drug Administration–approved type 2 5α-reductase inhibitor that affects the follicle, size, and amount of hair.
- Dutasteride is a type 1 and type 2 5α-reductase inhibitor used off-label to treat hair loss.

INTRODUCTION

For both men and women, having healthy hair denotes health, youth, and vitality. In mammals, hair serves a protective and evolutionary function. Although hair in humans may not be important for skin barrier protection from a biologic perspective, hair and pigment, or lack thereof, can have a significant impact on perceived social relevance as well emotional and psychological health. According to the American Hair Loss Association, more than $3.5 billion are spent each year by both men and women in the United States to treat hair loss. The practice of hair coloring has been documented since 1500 BC, and interest in hair restoration has not waned. The development of synthetic dyes for hair can be traced to the 1860s with the discovery of reactivity of p-phenylenediamine with air. Today, even with the advent of follicular unit extraction and various synthetic hair pigmentation regimens available to rejuvenate scalp hair, there remains a great demand for a product that could potentially halt, slow, or even reverse hair senescence. This article reviews the anatomy and physiology of hair growth and pigmentation as well as briefly reviewing the various biologic modifiers most commonly used.

ANATOMY OF THE HAIR FOLLICLE

Hair can grow individually, in groups of 2 to 3, or even at times in groups of 4 to 5. These groups are known as *follicular units*. Each individual hair shaft in the growth phase is composed of 3 main concentric regions: the medulla, cortex, and cuticle. The medulla comprises the innermost layer and is formed from transparent cells and air spaces that vary among different hair types. It is often difficult to identify on light microscopy and at times may be entirely absent. The cells comprising the medulla contain glycogen-rich vacuoles and medullary granules, which contain citrulline. The middle layer is called the cortex and is the business center of the hair shaft. The cortex is what comprises the bulk and lends the mechanical strength to the hair shaft; it is comprised of a highly structured protein, keratin, which is organized filaments made up of long, helical strands. The cells keratinize without forming granules through a process known as *trichilemmal*

Disclosure: None.
[a] Department of Otolaryngology Head and Neck Surgery, Division of Facial Plastic and Reconstructive Surgery, UCLA, 200 UCLA Medical Plaza, Suite 550, Los Angeles, CA 90095, USA; [b] Medcare Hospital, Dubai, United Arab Emirates
* Corresponding author. 221 West Pueblo Street, Santa Barbara, CA 93105.
E-mail address: apstl17@gmail.com

keratinization, as they move gradually upward from the hair matrix. The filamentous structure allows a single hair shaft to resist strain of up to 100 g, whereas the helical structure lends it elasticity. Therefore, the average full head of hair can hold more than 10 tons of weight. The groups of filaments form the cortex and are held together with disulfide, hydrogen, and salt bonds. This layer also has many important roles, such as storing the majority of the hair's moisture and housing the cells that lend pigment to the hair shaft. The number, distribution, and types of melanin granules contained in the cortex are what gives the hair fiber its pigment. Finally, the outer layer is known as the cuticle. This layer is composed of overlapping layers of 8 to 10 flat cells pointed outward and upward that interlock with the inner root sheath (IRS). When viewed under light electron microscopy, it has the appearance of roof shingles and is approximately 3 μm to 4 μm in thickness. When this layer is intact, it can last up to 6 years; it also reflects light and gives hair its shine and the appearance of good health.[1,2]

The hair follicle can be divided into 3 segments: lower, middle, and upper (**Figs. 1** and **2**). The lower segment is the area from the base of the follicle to the insertion of the arrector pili muscle and consists of the bulb and suprabulb regions. The bulb is comprised of the dermal papilla and the surrounding matrix. The papilla protrudes into

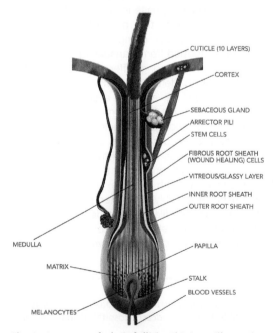

MEDULLA
MATRIX
MELANOCYTES

CUTICLE (10 LAYERS)
CORTEX
SEBACEOUS GLAND
ARRECTOR PILI
STEM CELLS
FIBROUS ROOT SHEATH (WOUND HEALING) CELLS
VITREOUS/GLASSY LAYER
INNER ROOT SHEATH
OUTER ROOT SHEATH
PAPILLA
STALK
BLOOD VESSELS

Fig. 1. Anatomy of a hair follicle. This is an illustration of the anatomy of a hair follicle and its associated adnexal structures. (*Courtesy of* Sajjad Khan, MD, Dubai, United Arab Emirates.)

the hair bulb and consists of an accumulation of egg-shaped mesenchymal cells, which direct hair growth. An abundance of melanin can be found within the melanophages that reside within the dermal papilla. The lower aspect of the papilla merges with the fibrous root sheath (FRS), which surrounds the hair follicle. It is the size of the papilla and the bulb that determines a hair's diameter. The matrix contains the hair's germination cells; this collection of peridermal cells divides rapidly and migrates upward to give rise to the hair shaft and internal root sheath. Melanin is transferred from the melanocytes found between the basal cells of the hair matrix to the cells, which make up the hair shaft. Hair pigmentation is determined by the quantity of melanin deposited to the growing hair shaft. The hair matrix cells give rise to 6 different types of cells that make up the different layers of the hair shaft and the IRS.[1,2]

The suprabulb region is the area between the hair bulb and the isthmus. It consists of the hair shaft, the IRS, the outer root sheath (ORS), vitreous layer (VL), and the FRS (see **Fig. 2**). The IRS serves to coat and support the hair shaft until it reaches the level of the isthmus, at which point it degenerates and exfoliates in the infundibular space. The IRS is composed of 3 concentric cell layers, which keratinize by forming trichohyalin granules (soft keratin): outer, middle, and inner. The outermost layer, also known as the Henle layer, keratinizes first. The middle layer, also referred to as the Huxley layer, keratinizes last. The cells of the innermost layer, also known as the IRS cuticle layer, keratinizes after the Henle layer. The cells of this innermost layer point downward and inward to interdigitate with the cells of the hair cuticle. Although these 3 layers are distinct, they keratinize relatively low in the hair follicle and become indistinguishable at higher levels, thereby enabling it to function as a single unit to cover the hair shaft. The ORS covers the IRS as it extends up from the matrix cells at the lower end of the hair bulb to the meatus of the sebaceous gland duct. It is thinnest at the bulb and thickest in the middle portion of the hair follicle. Only once the IRS disintegrates at the level of the isthmus does the ORS keratinize without forming granules. The ORS cells have a clear, vacuolated appearance due to the large amounts of glycogen. When the ORS reaches the level of the infundibulum, the keratinization changes to normal epidermal keratinization with formation of the granular cell layer and the stratum corneum. The vitreous (glossy) layer is an acellular, eosinophilic zone the surrounds the ORS. It is continuous with the epidermal

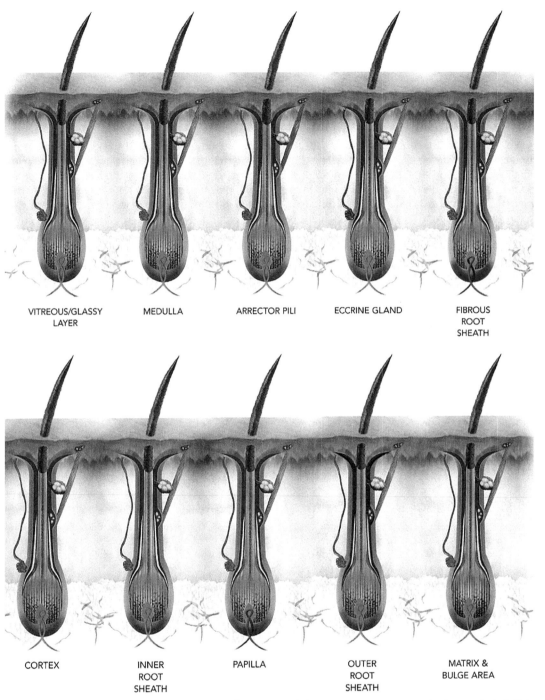

VITREOUS/GLASSY   MEDULLA   ARRECTOR PILI   ECCRINE GLAND   FIBROUS
LAYER   ROOT
                                                                                       SHEATH

CORTEX   INNER   PAPILLA   OUTER   MATRIX &
                ROOT   ROOT   BULGE AREA
                SHEATH   SHEATH

Fig. 2. Components of a hair follicle. This is an illustration of the unique components of a human hair follicle. (*Courtesy of* Sajjad Khan, MD, Dubai, United Arab Emirates.)

basement membrane. A distinguishing feature of catagen phase hairs is that the VR thickens and takes on a corrugated appearance. The FRS comprises the outermost layer of hair follicle and surrounds the VR. It consists of thickened collagen bundles that coat the entire hair follicle.

The FRS is continuous with the dermal papilla and the papillary dermis above it.[1,2]

The middle segment (isthmus) is short and spans from the insertion of the arrector pili muscle to the meatus of the sebaceous gland duct (see **Fig. 2**). The IRS fragments and exfoliates at this level, and at this point the ORS is fully keratinized via trichilemmal keratinization. The bulge region is difficult to appreciate on routine histology and is made up of densely packed cells with pluripotent capabilities encircled by the arrector pili muscle. Some believe that these stem cells that are residing in the bulge region are responsible for generating new hairs. Lastly, the upper segment of the hair follicle (infundibulum) extends from the meatus of the sebaceous gland duct to the follicular orifice. The epidermal surface lines the infundibulum and contains active pigmented melanocytes. The basal layer contains the inactive melanocytes, which are held in reserve and can become melanin-producing cells after injury to the skin. These cells then proliferate and migrate toward the regenerating upper portion of the ORS and the epidermis.[1,2]

When the hair transitions into the catagen phase (discussed later), the hair bulb keratinizes and turns into the club hair. This is then pushed upward to the surface by a column of thick and corrugated epithelial cells, which progressively shorten until it is reduced to a small saclike configuration, the secondary follicular germ. The dermal papilla also migrates upward, following the epithelial sac. During telogen, the secondary follicular germ and the dermal papilla form the telogen germinal unit, which gives rise to developing hair during anagen. The primary prenatal follicular germ unit regenerates the adnexal structures (ie, sebaceous and apocrine glands), whereas the telogen germinal unit does not.[1,2]

HAIR GROWTH CYCLE CHRONOLOGY

The average human has approximately 100,000 scalp hair shafts, each in varying degrees of the hair growth cycle. The average life cycle of a human hair shaft is approximately 3.5 years, and it grows approximately 0.05 in per month. There are 3 major phases of the hair growth cycle: anagen (growth), catagen (involution), and telogen (resting phase prior to being shed). The anagen phase lasts an average of 2 years to 7 years, the catagen phase approximately 2 weeks to 4 weeks, and the telogen phase approximately 3 months. Approximately 84% of scalp hairs are in the anagen phase, 1% to 2% in the catagen phase, and 10% to 15% in the telogen phase. Hair can be thick, long terminal hair or fine, short villous hair. In contrast, the eyelash hair follicles are shorter, lack an arrector pili muscle, and have a shorter hair cycle.[3]

Anagen refers to the active growth phase of hair, when the pigmented hair shafts are generated and the follicle reaches its maximal length and volume.

Approximately 85% to 90.6% of hair follicles are in this phase, which can last from 2 years to 6 years.[4,5] Catagen refers to the period of involution. During this phase, the epithelium of the lower follicle disintegrates and rises upwards with the papilla until it rests below the bulge zone, thereby forming the club hair. A streamer remains, which consists of the collapsed outermost layer (FRS). The hair follicle then enters a phase of relative quiescence, also known as telogen. This resting or dormant stage of the hair growth cycle is characterized by a marked decrease in proliferative and biochemical activity of the hair follicle. Although there is active hair growth or involution occurring, the existence of some baseline activity is believed important in intrinsic regulation of the hair cycle. During this phase, estrogen receptors are maximally expressed.[6] Exogen, also known as anagen stage IV, refers to the shedding of the hair shafts. These hairs are passively retained within the hair follicle but are distinguished from telogen clubs by the lack the cellular elements of the ORSs.[7]

HAIR PIGMENTATION

Unique hair color is a result of variations in the amount and type of melanin pigment production by cutaneous and follicular melanocytes. The biosynthesis of melanin occurs in intracellular organelles, known as melanosomes. The melanin produced by these melanosomes is then transferred from the melanocytes to the keratinocytes of skin and hair.

Two enzymes coded by the TYRP1 and DCT genes have been shown to biochemically alter the quality of melanin produced. Genes that have been shown to affect hair color include KITLG, IRF4, SLC24A4, and TPCN2.[8] The various stimulators and inhibitor of melanogenesis are listed in **Table 1**. Both melanocyte-stimulating hormone (MSH) and corticotropin are derived from proopiomelanocortin, which is synthesized by the pituitary gland and keratinocytes. MSH is believed to cause dispersion of the melanosomes and increase their melanogenic activity; α-MSH aids in the repairing of melanocytic DNA damage caused by exposure to UV radiation via reduction in UV-induced hydrogen peroxide formation, thereby maintaining melanosomal pH.

The loss of skin pigmentation from the skin epidermis can be indicative of the loss of pigment from hair follicles that have reached their terminal stage. During embryogenesis, the neural crest cells develop into hair follicle melanocytes. Hair follicles and sweat glands serve as reservoirs of melanocyte stem cells (MSCs). These melanocytes are

Table 1
Stimulators and inhibitors of melanogenesis

Stimulators	Inhibitors
MSH (α-MSH repairs DNA damage and maintains melanosomal pH)	Sphingolipids
	Bone morphogenetic protein 4
ACTH	Autoimmune processes (eg, vitiligo)
Endothelin-1	
Steel factor	
Prostaglandins and leukotrienes (inflammatory mediators)	
Neutrophins	
Basic fibroblast growth factor	
Nitric oxide	
Catecholamines	

Data from Talwar GP, Hasnain SE, Sarin SK. Textbook of biochemistry, biotechnology, allied and molecular medicine. 4th edition. Delhi (India): PHI Learning Private Limited; 2016. p. 277; with permission.

unable to produce melanin. These cells then undergo a life cycle of variable activity states that range from quiescent stem cells (melanoblasts), to proliferating, differentiating, and senescing terminally differentiated melanocytes. It is these mature melanocytes that produce melanin, but these cells are much more prone to cellular damage and apoptosis. Several factors, including microphthalmia-associated transcription factor, SOX10, PAX3, fibroblast growth factor-2, and endothelin-3, among others, are involved in committing early neural crest cells to the melanocyte lineage. Once committed to the melanocyte lineage, these cells then differentiate further into different melanocyte populations; several follicular melanocyte subpopulations exist in the adult human scalp and there is active turnover of these cells in accordance with the hair growth cycle.[9]

Hair color changes can be attributed to various cutaneous and systemic diseases as well as from exogenous influences. Hair darkening has been associated with Addison disease, neurodermatitis, and porphyria cutanea tarda. In contrast, hair lightening has been attributed to hyperthyroidism, acute extensive alopecia areata, vitiligo, and other genetic disorders, such as Werner syndrome, ataxia-telangiectasia (aka Louis-Bar Syndrome), and Waardenburg syndrome.[10] There are also several systemic drugs that have been known to induce hair color changes. Chloroquine, hydroxychloroquine, sunitinib, pazopanib, dasatinib, phenytoin, phenobarbital, tamoxifen, low-dose interferon, and mephenesin have all been reported to cause depigmentation

of hair. Imatinib, valproate, cisplatin, acitretin, and etretinate have been reported to cause either hyperpigmentation/repigmentation of gray hair or depigmentation, depending on the individual. Hyperpigmentation has been reported with the use of cyclosporine, indinavir, zidovudine, verapamil, and p-aminobenzoic acid. Additionally, different drug combinations can also result in color change. Cyclophosphamide, bleomycin, plus CCNU can change red hair to black; vincristine, bleomycin, and doxorubicin or vincristine alone can change black hair to red; cyclophosphamide, doxorubicin, and fluorouracil can change hair from blonde to dark brown, and a single dose of propofol, 140 mg, has been reported to turn blonde hair green within 2 days. Many, but not all, of these hair color changes have been reported to be reversible after cessation of drug administration.[11]

Hair pigment can be temporarily altered with the use of natural (ie, henna, indigo, berries, and other herbs) or synthetic hair coloring. Coating the hair cuticle or adding to the hair cuticle with color molecules gives temporary or semipermanent changes in hair pigmentation, whereas adding the color molecules to the deeper cortex layer yields more permanent alterations in hair color. Hydrogen peroxide is a key ingredient in the developer as it penetrates into the cortex layer and oxidizes the melanin, thereby removing color. Agents with a high pH (alkaline), such as ammonia, opens the cuticle to allow dye to enter the cortex and bind the keratin. Agents that are more acidic in the pH range of 4 to 5.5 seals the cuticle, thereby helping to lock in the new, desired color.

AGE-RELATED HAIR CHANGES

Genetics plays a large role in hair loss. Testosterone typically enters the papilla, ORS, and sebaceous gland cells where it is converted by 5α-reductase to dihydrotestosterone (DHT). DHT then binds to the androgen receptors and enters the nucleus where it binds the DNA and activates the production of proteins harmful to the follicle, thereby leading to disruption of the normal hair growth cycle. The overall growth cycle is altered in that the anagen phase is shortened, resulting in premature regression of the hair during its catagen and telogen phases. As new hair grows, there is a gradual reduction in the diameter of the hair follicle and the developing hair shaft. With each growth cycle, the anagen phase further shortens, resulting in a progressive miniaturization of hair and, eventually, hair loss. Genetics also plays a role in graying hair. In general, whites start to gray in their mid-30s, Asians in their late-30s, and Africans in their mid-40s. Those who develop graying hair in their 20s (or 30s for African Americans) are believed prematurely gray, likely due to a lack of pigment cell formation or to hydrogen buildup, which leads to hair bleaching. One of the byproducts of the hair growth process is the production of hydrogen peroxide, which is normally degraded by catalase. With aging, the decrement in catalase present in the cells allows for the accumulation of hydrogen peroxide and damage to the melanocytes.[1,12]

Additionally, the hair follicle is sensitive to cutaneous, systemic, and even environmental cues. These various inputs exert a modulatory effect on HF cycling, hair shaft growth, and hair pigmentation.[13] Age-related loss of hair pigmentation, also referred to as graying, has been linked to UV light and (genotoxic) reactive oxygen species (ROS)-induced cell damage. The hair follicle bulge harbors melanocyte stem cells, which then gives rise to mature melanocytes, which then synthesize and secrete hair pigment during Anagen. Several animal studies have demonstrated the effect of oxidant stress on hair coloring, and further studies have shown that graying human hair follicles contain melanocytes with accumulated oxidative stress and subsequent depletion of the stem cell population.[14] Melanotic bulbar melanocytes naturally express high levels of BCL-2, an antioxidant protein believed to help fight against melanogenesis and UV-A injury due to ROS formation. One animal study investigated the effect of BCL-2 in a mouse knockout model. Depilation-induced hair growth demonstrated a lack of visible melanin granules. It was hypothesized that increasing BCL-2 levels could enhance the antioxidant capacity of the hair follicle and thereby prevent hair graying. High levels of BCL-2, however, have been associated with the adverse effect of also increasing oncogenic potential.[15]

MODIFIERS OF HAIR GROWTH

There are many environmental and genetic factors that can affect the overall health of hair. The nutritional effects are summarized in **Table 2**. The various biologic modifiers are discussed later, and both the agent and its effects on hair are summarized in **Table 3**.

Minoxidil

The oral formulation of minoxidil was originally studied for its antihypertensive properties, but a notable side effect was that it caused generalized hypertrichosis. The topical application of minoxidil is often the first-line treatment for both men and women with hair loss. It is available over the counter as a solution (2% or 5%) or as foam (5%). The 2% solution is preferred for women because the 5% solution has been associated with an increased incidence of hypertrichosis outside of the treatment area.

Although minoxidil has been shown effective as a solo agent, multiple studies have demonstrated increased efficacy when used with other agents. The 5% topical minoxidil can be used in conjunction with oral finasteride, 1 mg, to enhance its overall antiandrogenetic alopecia effects. It can also be used once daily in combination with 0.01% tretinoin, which has been found more effective than the use of just 5% minoxidil twice daily; application of the 5% topical solution or foam resulted in an increase in hair regrowth in 45% of male subjects.

How minoxidil asserts its effects on the growth of the hair follicle is poorly understood. Initially it was suggested that minoxidil caused vasodilation of the follicle cell vasculature, but a recent study by Shorter and colleagues[16] suggested that it may affect the regulation of one of the 2 ATP-sensitive potassium channels present in human follicular dermal papillae, SUR2. Additional animal and human studies have demonstrated that there is an increase in hair weight with use of minoxidil, which suggests that the therapeutic effect may be due to increasing the diameter of hair or the hair follicle.[17]

Finasteride (Propecia [Merck & Co])

Another commonly prescribed agent for male and female hair loss is finasteride. This type 2 5α-reductase inhibitor is Food and Drug Administration (FDA) approved in 1997 for the treatment of male pattern hair loss and is orally administered at the optimal dose of 1 mg daily. Use of finasteride, 1 mg, resulted in a 64% decrease in median scalp DHT compared with placebo and a 71% decrease in median serum DHT levels.[18] After several months of therapy, patients report increased hair diameter, growth rate, and, to a lesser extent, increased hair counts.

Dutasteride (Avodart)

The agent dutasteride (Avodart [GSK]) was approved by the FDA in 2002 for the treatment of benign prostatic hypertrophy, but due to its potent antiandrogenic effects has also been used off-label for the treatment of hair loss. It is both a type 1 and type 2 5α-reductase inhibitor. A study comparing the effects of dutasteride to finasteride and placebo demonstrated that a daily dose of dutasteride, 2.5 mg, was statistically superior to finasteride in increasing hair counts.[19]

Platelet-Rich Plasma

Platelet-rich plasma (PRP) is prepared by concentrating the red blood cells and separating it from

Table 2
Nutritional effects on hair growth and health.

Nutritional Agent	Effect on Hair	Associated Food(s)
Water	Moisture	8 glasses/d
Iron	Carries oxygen to hair and promotes growth	Chicken Spinach Lentils Beef liver
Vitamin A	Antioxidant reduces free radicals and inflammation	Carrots Spinach Sweet potatoes Kale
B-complex vitamins (biotin, niacin, and cobalamine)	Restore shine and thickness to hair strands	Peanuts Sweet potatoes Almonds Eggs Chicken Sardines Tuna Whole grains
Vitamin D	Important for hair follicle cycling	Mushrooms Beef liver Salmon Low-fat diary Whole grains
Vitamin C	Helps grow and strengthen hair, also absorbs iron	Broccoli Bell peppers Strawberries Pineapple Oranges
Vitamin E	Strengthens hair, improves volume and circulation	Almonds Peanuts Spinach
Silica	Strengthens hair	Green beans Oats Cucumber Bell peppers
Copper	Essential for health of hair; needed to produce antioxidant superoxide dismutase	Sesame seeds Legumes Seaweed Cashews Animal liver
Selenium	Important for healthy scalp	Mushrooms Shrimp Whole grains Tuna fish Brazil nuts
Potassium	Helps maintain hair moisture and healthy pH	Sweet potatoes Bananas Yogurt Spinach Coconut water Swiss chard
Magnesium	Essential for proper hair growth and strengthens hair	Swiss chard Pumpkin seeds Spinach Dark chocolate Beet greens

(continued on next page)

Table 2
(continued)

Nutritional Agent	Effect on Hair	Associated Food(s)
Omega-3 fatty acids	Prevents inflammation and promotes hair growth	Salmon Chia Flax Sardine fish Walnuts Beef
Calcium	A key component of hair growth	Low-fat dairy Spinach Sardine fish

This chart summarizes the nutritious foods and their effect on hair. Biotin, also known as vitamin B7, is not listed but is believed to play an important role in the health and growth of skin, hair, and nails. A deficiency in this vitamin is believed to contribute to hair loss

the platelets and plasma. When the concentrated platelets are activated, they release growth factors that have been shown beneficial in the treatment of hair loss. It is believed that the platelet growth factors may reverse the miniaturization process and result in restoration of the normal hair cycle. A recent review determined an average of 3 injection treatments are needed to achieve some benefit.[20] For more information, see Karam W. Badran and Jordan P. Sand's article, "Platelet Rich Plasma for Hair Loss: Review of Methods and Results," in this issue.

Latisse (Bimatoprost Ophthalmic Solution 0.03%)

Originally prescribed to treat open-angle glaucoma and ocular hypertension, the agent bimatoprost ophthalmic solution, 0.03% (Latisse) lowers the intraocular pressure by increasing the outflow of aqueous humor via the trabecular meshwork and the uveoscleral routes. It was incidentally noted that the patient using this medication also developed longer eyelashes. The exact mechanism of action by which eyelash growth is

Table 3
Biologics and effects on hair. This chart summarizes the various biologic agents that modify hair growth

Agent	Mechanism of Effect
Minoxidil	Vasodilation of follicle vasculature. May affect ATP-sensitive K^+ channels in human follicular dermal papillae (SUR2). May result in increased hair follicle diameter.
Finasteride	Type 2 5α-reductase inhibitor.
Dutasteride	Type 1 and type 2 5α-reductase inhibitor
PRP	Platelet growth factors may reverse the miniaturization process and results in restoration of normal hair cycle.
Latisse	A synthetic prostaglandin $F_{2\alpha}$ analog that prolongs anagen phase of eyelash hair follicles.
Aldactone/spironolactone	Blocks the receptor binding of DHT. Spironolactone slows adrenal gland and ovarian production of androgens.
PTHrP antagonist	Promotes hair follicle activation.
Cimetidine	Histamine blocker and also blocks DHT from binding the follicular receptor sites.
Cyproterone acetate	Blocks the binding of DHT to its receptors. Available in Europe only.
Oral contraceptives	Decreases ovarian androgen production, thus used to treat androgenetic alopecia in women.

stimulated is unknown, but it is believed to prolong the anagen phase of eyelash hair follicles. Bimatoprost is a synthetic prostaglandin $F_{2\alpha}$ analog.[21] An irreversible side effect noted in 1% to 2% of glaucoma patients using this medication is iris hyperpigmentation (increased brown pigmentation), in addition to possible reversible darkening of the eyelid skin.

ALTERNATIVE TREATMENT OPTIONS
Spironolactone (Aldactone)

Spironolactone (Aldactone [Pfizer]) is a popular potassium-sparing diuretic used in the treatment of hypertension but is also an antiandrogen. Spironolactone slows down adrenal gland and ovarian production of androgens. Additionally, it also blocks the binding of DHT to its androgenetic receptor.

Parathyroid Hormone–Related Peptide Antagonists

Two key studies published in 1994 demonstrated in vitro and in vivo that parathyroid hormone–related peptide (PTHrP) antagonists promoted follicular activation whereas PTHrP agonists inhibited hair follicle formation. A subsequent study investigated 2 different antagonists and showed that these increased anagen hair follicles at 2 weeks.[22]

Cimetidine

Cimetidine (Tagmet) is a well-known histamine blocker used to treat gastrointestinal ulcers. Cimetadine, however, also has a powerful antiandrogenic effect and has been shown to block DHT from binding the follicle receptor sites. This agent has been used to treat hirsutism in women, and its use in initial studies to treat androgenic alopecia has shown promise.

Cyproterone Acetate

The agent cyproterone acetate is not available in the United States but is available in Europe. It has been used to reduce sex drive in men and has also been used to treat severe hirsutism in women. Cyproterone acetate blocks the binding of DHT to its receptors but, due to its long-term side effects, is considered a last resort for treating female pattern hair loss. When combined with ethinylestradiol, it is sold under the brand names Diane-35 and Diane-50 (Ocean Pharmaceutical) in Europe as a contraceptive agent.

Estrogen/Progesterone

Estrogen/progesterone is prescribed to women in menopause as hormone replacement therapy in the form of pills or cream and is used as a systemic form of treatment of androgenetic alopecia in menopausal women or in those with low hormone levels.

Oral Contraceptives

Birth control pills exert their effects by decreasing the production of ovarian androgens; therefore, birth control pills may be used to treat androgenetic alopecia in women. Low androgen index birth control pills are used to treat hair loss. High androgen index birth control pills are avoided because use of these can trigger hair loss.

REFERENCES

1. Khan S. Guide to hair. Dubai: Dr. Sajjad Khan Publisher; 2017.
2. Alaiti S, Meyers A, Talavera F, et al. Hair anatomy. Available at: https://emedicine.medscape.com/article/835470. Accessed December 13, 2017.
3. Paus R, Burgoa I, Platt CI, et al. Biology of the eyelash hair follicle: an enigma in plain sight. Br J Dermatol 2016;174:741–52.
4. Mulinari-Brenner F, Neto FJ, Ross FMB, et al. Morphometry of normal scalp hair follicles. An Bras Dermatol 2006;81(1):46–52.
5. Wosicka H, Cal K. Targeting to the hair follicles: current status and potential. J Dermatol Sci 2010;57: 83–9.
6. Paus R, Foitzik K. In search of the "hair cycle clock": a guided tour. Differentiation 2004;72:489–511.
7. Van neste D, Leroy T, Conil S. Exogen hair characterization in human scalp. Skin Res Technol 2007;13(4): 436–43.
8. Sturm R. Molecular genetics of human pigmentation diversity. Hum Mol Genet 2009;18(R1):R9–17.
9. Commo S, Bernard BA. Melanocyte subpopulation turnover during the human hair cycle: an immunohistochemial study. Pigment Cell Res 2000;13(4): 253–9.
10. Francesco R, De Simone C, DelRegno L, et al. Drug-induced hair colour changes. Eur J Dermatol 2016; 26(6):531–6.
11. Ricci F, De Simone C, Del Regno L, et al. Drug-induced hair colour changes. Eur J Dermatol 2016; 26(6):531–6.
12. Westgate GE, Botchkareva NV, Tobin DJ. The biology of hair diversity. Int J Cosmet Sci 2013; 35(4):329–36.
13. Paus R, Lagan EA, Vidali S, et al. Neuroendocrinology of the hair follicle: principles and clinical perspectives. Trends Mol Med 2014;20(10):559–70.
14. Geyfman M, Andersen B. Clock genes, hair growth and aging. Aging 2010;2(3):122–8.
15. Selberg M. Age-induced hair greying – the multiple effects of oxidative stress. Int J Cosmet Sci 2013; 35:532–8.

16. Shorter K, Farjo NP, Picksley SM, et al. Human hair follicles contain two forms of ATP-sensitive potassium channels, only one of which is sensitive to minoxidil. FASEB J 2008;22(6):1725–36.

17. Nusbaum AG, Rose PT, Nusbaum BP. Nonsurgical therapy for hair loss. Facial Plast Surg Clin North Am 2013;21:335–42.

18. Drake L, Hordinsky M, Fiedler V. The effects of finasteride on scalp skin and serum androgen levels in men with androgenetic alopecia. J Am Acad Dermatol 1999;41:550–4.

19. Olsen EA, Hordinsky M, Whiting D, et al. The importance of dual 5alpha-reductase inhibition in the treatment of male pattern hair loss: results of a randomized placebo-controlled study of dutasteride versus finasteride. J Am Acad Dermatol 2006;55(6):1014–23.

20. Sand JP, Nabili V, Kochhar A, et al. Platelet-rich plasma for the aesthetic surgeon. Facial Plast Surg 2017;33:437–43.

21. Cohen J. Enhancing the growth of natural eyelashes: the mechanism of bimatoprost-induced eyelash growth. Dermatol Surg 2010;36:1361–71.

22. Robert C. Gensure. Parathyoid hormone-related peptide and the hair cycle – is it the agonists or the antagonists that cuase hair growth? Exp Dermatol 2014;23:865–7.

Stem Cells in Dermatology and Anti-aging Care of the Skin

Amy Forman Taub, MD[a,b,c],*, Kim Pham, MPH[d,1]

KEYWORDS

- Stem cells • Anti-microbial peptide • Defensin • Anti-aging skin care • Pore reduction
- Epidermal thickness • Melanin • Wrinkles

KEY POINTS

- A key hallmark to skin aging is the exhaustion or dysregulation of the endogenous stem cell population, which aids in maintaining tissue homeostasis and repair of injured tissues.
- Specific stem cell populations located in hair follicles perform many of these functions for the skin and are activated by defensin peptides, which are released by neutrophils during skin wounding.
- Exogenous defensins in a skin care formulation have been shown in published studies to be effective for some clinical signs of skin aging.

INTRODUCTION

Since the discovery of multipotent stem cells by Till and McCulloch in 1961,[1] further elucidation of stem cells' functions have been identified as both facilitating development of new cells and maintaining homeostasis of current normal cells. The activity of stem cells is stimulated by the start of tissue dysfunction. Several applications using these functions have been implemented in medicine already: reestablishing the hematopoietic lineage via bone marrow transplantation,[2] development of stem-cell based therapy for type 1 diabetes[3,4] and retinitis pigmentosa,[5] and using stem cells to advance the cure for spinal cord injury.[6] One important application of stem cell biology is how these cells can be used in the context of aging and age-related dysfunctions. During aging, DNA accumulates damage, impairing protein homeostasis, cell function and communication, as well as normal organ physiology.[7] Another key hallmark to aging is the exhaustion or dysregulation of the endogenous stem cell population, which aids in maintaining tissue homeostasis and repair of injured tissues. Because aging is so intimately tied to stem cell integrity, one of the major goals of stem cell biology and regenerative medicine is how one can use these cells to reverse aging and the associated dysfunctions that come with it.

Stem cells are undifferentiated or partially differentiated cells that are capable of dividing and generating differentiated and proliferative cells (**Fig. 1**). Stem cells range from pluripotent cells that are found in the inner cell mass of pre-implantation blastocysts or isolated from other sources to unipotent progenitors such as fetal tissues, birth-associated tissues, or adult tissues. Several advances have been made to apply the unique traits of this variety of stem

Disclosure: Dr A.F. Taub has been paid by Medicell Technologies for research conducted as well as honoraria for speaking. She also has a small equity in the company. She was not paid to produce this paper. K. Pham was paid an honorarium to assist in this publication.

[a] Department of Dermatology, Northwestern University, Medical School, Chicago, IL, USA; [b] Advanced Dermatology, 275 Parkway Drive, Suite 521, Lincolnshire, IL 60069, USA; [c] Advanced Dermatology, Glencoe, IL, USA; [d] University of Wisconsin, School of Medicine and Public Health, Madison, WI, USA

[1] Present address: 2355 University Avenue Apartment 2015, Madison, WI 53726.

* Corresponding author. 275 Parkway Drive, Suite 521, Lincolnshire, IL 60069.

E-mail address: drtaub@advdermatology.com

Facial Plast Surg Clin N Am 26 (2018) 425–437
https://doi.org/10.1016/j.fsc.2018.06.004

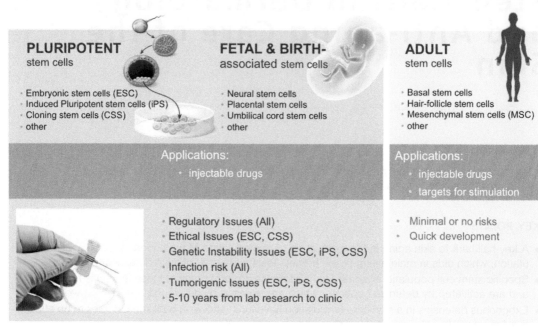

Fig. 1. Types of human stem cells.

cell types. These include establishment of an embryonic stem cell line via in vitro fertilization, the reprogramming of differentiated adult cells to induced pluripotent stem cells (iPSC), and the generation of cloning stem cells (somatic nuclear transfer stem cells). Other strategies include the creation of parthenogenetic stem cells, isolation of stem cells from fetal tissues (including neural stem cells or retinal progenitor cells), and separation of birth-associated stem cell populations including cord blood stem cells or placental stem cells. Although these different modes of pluripotent and fetal stem cells provide great potential for treating aging and age-related diseases, there are several associated disadvantages. Pluripotent and fetal stem cells may be tumorigenic,[8] possess genetic instability,[9] and are often tied to ethical and regulatory debate.[10] Even though iPSCs bypass the ethical issues of embryonic stem cells, they still possess the same mutations and damage that the donor cells had, which can decrease its ability to proliferate and respond to its respective niche.[11] Stem cells isolated from birth-associated tissues have limited ability to proliferate and limited directions of differentiation, and therefore therapeutic potential of areas of their applications is rudimental.[12] An alternative method that is being explored is the use of pharmaceuticals to modulate endogenous stem cell populations to leverage their respective mechanism of cell signaling and communication.

One such example is the use of CBP/Catenin antagonist, ICG-001, that acts more selectively than retinol by shifting the balance of cell division to asymmetric division and thus more differentiation.[13] With more alternative methods emerging in regenerative medicine, several other advances that target the individual's stem cells could provide the means for dealing with age-related dysfunctions such as skin aging.

DERMATOLOGIC STEM CELLS

There has been great interest in understanding the regulation and coordination of the stem cells found within the skin in order to repair aged skin (**Fig. 2**). Through wound healing and genetic knock out experiments, several stem cell populations have been elucidated in the skin that have applications to regenerative medicine.[14,15] Within the epidermis lay basal epidermal stem cells that proliferate and maintain epidermal turnover and homeostasis.[14] Other stem cells that are involved in transient repair of skin wounds (although they do not contribute skin's homeostasis on a daily basis) are hair follicle stem cells.[15] These follicular-based stem cells include *Lrig1*+ stem cells (residing in the junctional zone of the hair follicle and contributing to the infundibulum), *Gli1*+ stem cells (maintaining sebaceous glands), and *Lgr6*+ stem cells (acting as skin's master stem cells).[14,16] The *Lgr6*+ cells are termed "master" cells

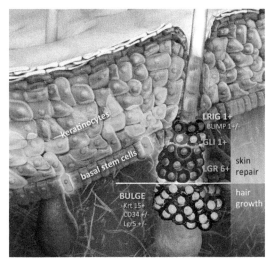

LRIG 1+
BLIMP 1+/-
GLI 1+
LGR 6+
keratinocytes
basal stem cells
skin repair
hair growth
BULGE
Krt 15+
CD34 +/-
Lgr5 +/-

Fig. 2. Dermatologic stem cells. Basal stem cells support epidermal turnover and keratinocyte renewal. Bulge stem cells in hair follicle (Wnt-dependent cells) are primarily responsible for hair growth because of their ability to respond to Wnt, the major hair growth signal. Stem cells located above bulge of hair follicle (Wnt-independent cells) enable epidermis repair in wounds and support other functions than hair growth skin's functions; these cells can not contribute into hair growth because they have no Wnt receptors and therefore unable to respond to hair growth signal. (*From* Taub A, Bucay V, Keller G, et al. Multicenter, double-blind, vehicle-controlled clinical trial of an alpha and beta defensin-containing anti-aging skin care regimen with clinical, histopathologic, immunohistochemical, photographic, and ultrasound evaluation. J Drugs Dermatol 2018;17(4):426–41; with permission.)

because they are the ones that create the entire epidermis and appendages early in utero.[17] Although these different cell types are compartmentalized in their respective niche, some are able to contribute to different tissues at different times to maintain sebaceous glands and interfollicular epidermis or aid in wound repair.[14] Moreover, these stem cells are less susceptible to damage via aging[18] (because they lay dormant for much of life until signals of distress stimulate them to reproduce), thus garnering interest in further experimentations concerning their regenerative capacity.

Epidermal Stem Cells

Within the *stratum basale* are basal cells that act as the stem cells for epidermal homeostasis. Although further understanding is needed about these cells and how they proliferate, 2 major models are proposed about the mode in which

these cells divide. In the epidermal proliferative unit model,[19] a single basal cell acts as the source of self-renewal and proliferation per unit.[19] With this model, the entire epidermis can be considered a collection of epidermal proliferative units each marked by the presence of a single basal cell. On the contrary, the Committed Progenitor model proposes that basal cells divide stochastically, resulting in 2 differentiated daughter cells, more basal cells, or one of each.[20] In order to reconcile these 2 prevailing models, a third model was proposed to integrate aspects of the two. This model argues that the existence of these 2 modes of division allow the maintenance of the epidermis and also prompt wound healing when necessary.[21]

Hair Follicle Stem Cells

An important group of stem cells to the skin is found within the hair follicle. Most stem cells in the follicle express Shh with some, such as *Lgr6+* and *Lrig1+*, exhibiting Sox9 expression.[16,17,22,23] Despite a similar development, different stem cell populations are confined to a discrete section of the hair follicle, and under physiologic conditions, they have a specified regenerative function, whether it is hair cycling or sebaceous gland maintenance.[24] In addition, hair follicle stem cells do not contribute to the epidermis during normal physiologic events,[14] which could be due to minimal cross-talk between compartments as well as a gradient of responsiveness to different molecular cues. On circumstances such as wounding, certain populations are mobilized to help reepithelialize the skin or aid in hair follicle neogenesis.[25,26]

Bulge cells are slow-cycling hair follicle stem cells that are positive for *Keratin 15 (K15)* expression.[27] Normally, these cells remain quiescent but can engage in cycling of anagen hair follicles. Bulge cells can also upregulate *Lhx2* to temporarily reconstitute interfollicular epidermis after injury.[28] Progeny of these cells provide rapid reepithelialization of the wounded skin that is later replaced by epidermally derived keratinocytes. A second stem cell population in the hair follicle is *Lrig1+* cells that exist above bulge cells in the junctional zone. These cells provide for the maintenance of the infundibulum and also sebaceous gland structures.[29] Like bulge cells, these cells can also engage in wound healing by producing epidermally fated clones. However, unlike bulge stem cells, *Lrig1+* progeny lasts longer in the epidermis and continues to proliferate postwounding.[15] Located above the hair bulge is another stem cell population of note called *Lgr6+* cells, which are similar to Lrig1+ stem cells. In contrast to other populations that normally maintain one aspect of dermatologic homeostasis, this population is multipotent and can provide cells to the epidermis or the sebaceous gland in the absence of skin injury.[30] In the event of wounding though, Lgr6+ cells also aid in long-lasting repair of the epidermis.

Sebaceous and Sweat Gland Stem Cells

Both the sebaceous and sweat glands are appendages that aid in maintenance of the skin. Sweat glands provide thermoregulation, excretion, and immune function, whereas sebaceous glands lubricate the skin. In the sweat gland are suprabasal progenitors that can create sweat-producing luminal cells.[31] Within the gland are also ductal cells that maintain ductal openings on the skin and can also regenerate the epidermis surrounding the sweat gland after tissue injury. As for sebaceous glands, Blimp1+ cells produce sebocyte progenitors.[31]

LGR6+ STEM CELLS: THE SKIN'S MASTER STEM CELLS

As mentioned earlier, Lgr6+ cells are multipotent cells found within the hair follicle above the bulge that actively cycle to contribute to the epidermis and sebaceous gland.[32] When investigating the development of these cells, Snippert and colleagues[17] observed that Lgr6+ is first expressed embryonically in the early placode (embryonic structures that give rise to structures such as hair follicles and teeth) and remains expressed during hair development. Eventually, expression spreads from the hair follicle to the interfollicular epidermis until it becomes later restricted to the central isthmus above the hair bulge in adult skin. Thus, Lgr6+ cells are considered primitive epidermal stem cells by establishing the epithelial placode, confirming their multipotency in adult skin.[33] This multipotency was later observed in a transplantation study in nude mice and wounded skin where Lgr6+ cells can form all skin lineages.[34] In addition, through lineage tracing in the wound, it was also confirmed that Lgr6+ cells aid in long-term wound healing.[14,17]

Lgr6+ cell's involvement in wound healing, as well as its multipotency, are 2 key interests in the study of skin aging and regeneration. It is known that Lgr6+ cells can migrate into the wound center to aid in reepithelialization.[33] Activation, migration, and eventual proliferation of these cells are triggered by cytokines that are secreted by neutrophils for pathogen defense.[33] Interestingly, implanted Lgr6+ stem cells also aided in hair follicle neogenesis within wounds 10 to 15 days postwounding and genes commonly expressed (such as vascular endothelial growth factor [VEGF], hepatocyte growth factor, and tumor necrosis factor) in wound healing were upregulated.[34] Even with these limitations, Lgr6+ cells remain of great interest in their role in establishing various epidermal cell lines postwounding. Elucidation of the development of these cells, how they remain localized in adult hair follicles, and wound-induced

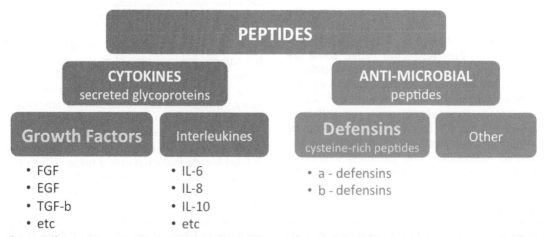

Fig. 3. Defensins are not growth factors. Defensins are a group of antimicrobial peptides that are functionally and structurally different from growth factors. (*From* Taub A, Bucay V, Keller G, et al. Multi-center, double-blind, vehicle-controlled clinical trial of an alpha and beta defensin-containing anti-aging skin care regimen with clinical, histopathologic, immunohistochemical, photographic, and ultrasound evaluation. J Drugs Dermatol 2018;17(4):426–41; with permission.)

recruitment are topics of interest for skin regeneration and aging.

DEFENSINS

Defensins are a group of antimicrobial peptides that are functionally and structurally different from growth factors (**Fig. 3**). β-defensins are peptides secreted by the skin epithelium and are of importance to *Lgr6+*-mediated skin healing. This peptide comes from a family shared with α-defensins that serves multiple functions. First, β-defensins provide innate immunity by deterring microbial colonization on the skin surface.[35] They also enhance tight junctions while bringing into tight junction structures one of their key components, claudin proteins, thereby reducing paracellular permeability of the skin epidermis (the transfer of substances across an epithelium by passing through the intercellular space between the cells) and eventually preventing transepidermal water loss.[36] A third function of β-defensin is to induce wound healing by recruiting *Lgr6+* stem cells to create new basal stem cells in the wound and thus stimulate the creation of new keratinocytes in the wound bed[33] (**Fig. 4**).

One application proposed and studied for this peptide is the use of intestinal α-defensins on skin to stimulate *Lgr6+* stem cells. Lough and colleagues[33] found that healing was enhanced in murine skin wounds on induction of α-defensin 5 as observed by rapid wound closure and hair follicle neogenesis within the wound bed. This enhancement of healing was mediated by the recruitment of *Lgr6+* cells. Because of these results, use of α-defensins would be particularly useful in large-scale wounds or burns where the local stem cell niche is removed and β-defensins are no longer present on the skin surface to induce wound healing.[33] In addition, because *Lgr6+* is involved in new keratinocyte production, α-defensins could also have applications in reversing skin aging.[33]

AGING AND APPLICATIONS

Aging is considered the decline or deterioration of physiologic functions often attributed to accumulated alterations in the genome, decreased telomere length, protein and cellular damage, increased inflammation and cell senescence, exhaustion of endogenous stem cell populations, and issues with intercellular communication.[7] Although not exhaustive, all of these molecular and cellular mechanisms can work in concert with one another to accelerate the process of aging but also attenuate aging if repaired. Moreover, these proposed molecular characteristics of aging may actually be used by the body as a form of beneficial repair that ultimately becomes detrimental and compromises the integrity of target tissues or organs.[7]

Although not comprehensive, some of the major sources that lead to skin aging include ultraviolet (UV) damage, environmental insults, inflammation, and an increase in reactive oxidative species in comparison to antioxidant.[37,38] Overall, the damage created by these different sources leads to deterioration and damage of the epidermal tissue as well as the loss of collagen and elastin in the dermis.[39] Aging is also considered the cause of a decrease in epidermal thickness and growth factors available in the skin.[39] Although they may seem as distinct events, aging and wound healing have commonalities due to similar genetic and cellular pathways, which compensate and replenish. During the initial phase of wound healing, inflammation arises via reactive oxygen species.[39] In the same manner, skin aging is often associated with the increase in the presence of reactive oxidative species.[39] Although there are several other commonalities between the two, both aging and wound healing involve a departure from fetal skin repair, where skin is scarless and maintains normal collagen integrity.

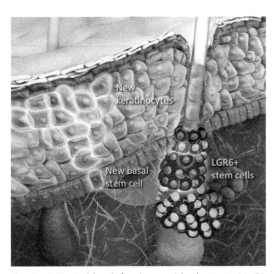

Fig. 4. Activated by defensin peptide dormant *Lgr6+* stem cells create new basal stem cells and thus stimulate the creation of new keratinocytes. (*From* Taub A, Bucay V, Keller G, et al. Multi-center, double-blind, vehicle-controlled clinical trial of an alpha and beta defensin-containing anti-aging skin care regimen with clinical, histopathologic, immunohistochemical, photographic, and ultrasound evaluation. J Drugs Dermatol 2018;17(4):426–41; with permission.)

During fetal wound healing, repair of full-thickness wounds results in the full restoration of the epidermis, dermis, hair follicles, sebaceous glands, and sweat glands without scarring.[40] In contrast, adult wound healing is associated with fibrosis and an altered composition of the skin surface that is marked by dense collagen networks and loss of structures such as hair follicles. The different responses of these 2 processes have been studied, and although more needs to be understood, it seems that fetal wound healing uses different genetic and inflammatory responses along with different intercellular signaling. One example that highlights this change in responses between fetal and adult wound healing is the upregulation of fibroblast growth factor 2 during repair in fetal wounds but not in adult wounds, which inhibits the fibrosis response that is seen in adult wound healing.[41]

The insights from wounding studies demonstrate the gaps observed in adult skin healing and provide mechanisms to recapitulate the same processes seen in fetal skin regeneration. Elucidations of these different mechanisms have potential applications in the reversal and delay in skin aging. One treatment that has been proposed is the use of mesenchymal stem cells in the placenta or umbilical cord.[42] Some of the advantages for the use of these extraembryonic cells are their similarity to embryonic stem cells, multipotency, and higher efficacy in regeneration when compared with adult-derived mesenchymal stem cells. Despite these benefits, there are issues with controlling differentiation direction that these cells will take, and little information is known about how mesenchymal cells participate in fetal wound healing.[41]

Another growing field in terms of skin therapies is the use of growth factors to induce keratinocyte and collagen proliferation. Growth factors are regulatory peptides that participate in cell to cell signaling as well as intracellular signaling such as chemotaxis, division, and differentiation.[43] These proteins can be produced by fibroblasts, platelets, keratinocytes, and immunomodulatory cells. In comparison to other peptides that aid in intercellular signaling, these proteins are defined by possessing a targeted response. This is beneficial during post–skin wounding where these growth factors can diffuse into the wound bed and aid in repair by inducing collagen proliferation, promoting angiogenesis, stimulating cell migration and division, and reducing local inflammation.[44]

The understanding of growth factors in aging skin was elucidated through the studies of skin wound healing.[45] Here, growth factors were found to act in repair by mediating in the inflammatory, granulation, and remodeling stages seen after wounding. In this case, multiple growth factors such as VEGF, transforming growth factor beta (TGF-β), and interleukin 8 coordinate to resolve the wound.[45] One of the main goals seen during this event is for growth factors to reestablish the extracellular matrix and ensure collagen and elastin production is made.[46] With that in mind, the function and mechanism of growth factors in wounds can be translated in its therapeutic use to skin aging where growth factor count is diminished and the aged skin possesses a reduced collagen network. Specifically, growth factors can decelerate aging by stimulating keratinocytes to produce more growth factors that can promote collagen synthesis as well as keratinocyte division.[39]

Although growth factors have been used successfully to treat skin aging,[39] there is still a need to further understand which components are necessary for efficacy and to clarify some controversies over safety. Initial growth factors introduced into cosmeceuticals were derived from plants or plant stem cell sources. For example, kinetin has been shown to be effective in improving the appearance of aging skin due to its natural ability to prevent plant leaves from drying out and withering. Using topical 0.1% kinetin, patients saw a 26% increase in the ability of skin to retain moisture in 24 weeks.[47] Plant (including apple) stem cell extracts is a "soup" of plant-originated proteins, cytokines, and growth factors. This mixture contains undefined molecules with nonspecificity and low efficacy.[48] Because of the lack of specificity, this treatment can activate a wide array of cells, which could be deleterious if unregulated. Moreover, plant stem cells act on the host's old basal stem cells that may still possess the genetic alterations and insults seen with the accumulative effects of internal aging and photoaging. Since then, other applications of growth factor therapy have been created, such as the use of conditioned medium growth factors.[39] The example of the secretome of cultured mesenchymal stem cells is shown in **Table 1**. Here, there is more efficacy on age reversal or deceleration compared with plant stem cells, but like its predecessor, this strategy contains undefined growth factors that are nonspecific and only target aged cells of the skin.[49] More than a decade ago, when first growth factor products were just introduced to the market it was an authentic revolutionary approach. Cancer research has unearthed concerns relating to the use of undefined compositions of growth factors (conditioned media) for skin care purposes.[50–56] For example, TGF-β is present in most of the

Table 1
Trophic and immunomodulatory factors secreted by cultured mesenchymal stem cells

Effect	Molecule
Antiapoptotic	VEGF
	HGF
	IGF-I
	Stanniocalcin-1
	TGF-b
	bFGF
	GM-CSF
Immunomodulatory	PGE-2
	TGF-b
	HGF
	mpCCL2
	IDO
	iNOS
	HLA-G5
	LIF
Antiscarring	bFGF
	HGF
	Adrenomedullin (?)
Supportive	SCF
	LIF
	IL-6
	M-CSF
	SDF-1
	Angiopoietin-1
Angiogenic	bFGF
	VEGF
	PIGF
	MCP-1
	IL-6
	Extracellular matrix molecules
Chemoattractant	CCL2 (MCP-1)
	CCL3 (MIP-1a)
	CCL4 (MIP-1b)
	CCL5 (RANTES)
	CCL7 (MCP-3)
	CCL20 (MIP-3a)
	CCL26 (eotaxin-3)
	CX3CL1 (fractalkine)
	CXCL5 (ENA-78)
	CXCL11 (i-TAC)
	CXCL1 (GROa)
	CXCL2 (GROb)
	CXCL8 (IL-8)
	CCL10 (IP-10)
	CXCL12 (SDF-1)

Abbreviations: bFGF, basic fibroblast growth factor; ENA-78, epithelial-derived neutrophil-activating peptide 78; GM-CSF, granulocyte-macrophage colony-stimulating factor; HGF, hepatocyte growth factor; HLA-G5, human leukocyte antigen-G; IDO, indoleamine 2,3-deoxygenase; IGF, insulin-like growth factor; IL-6, interleukin 6; iNOS, induced nitric oxide synthase; IP-10, interferon γ-induced protein 10; i-TAC, interferon-inducible T-cell alpha chemoattractant; LIF, leukemia inhibitory factor; MCP-1, monocyte chemoattractant protein-1; MIP-3a, macrophage inflammatory protein; PGE-2, prostaglandin E2; PIGF, placental growth factor; SDF-1, stromal cell-derived factor 1; SCF, stem cell factor.

From Meirelles Lda S, Fontes AM, Covas DT, et al. Mechanisms involved in the therapeutic properties of mesenchymal stem cells. Cytokine Growth Factor Rev 2009;20(5–6):419–27; with permission.

conditioned media.[50,51] Multiple cancer research studies show that TGF-β is a very potent trigger of the cancer-related pathways.[52,53,56] For example, TGF-β overproduction, as a driver of the fibrotic process of chronic phases of inflammatory diseases, precedes tumor formation and prepares a favorable microenvironment for cancer cells.[54,55]

Because of these drawbacks, more well-defined growth factors were the next step in skin aging therapy. In comparison to the preceding 2 treatments, there is a defined growth factor that is given for treatment, leading to greater control of application and results.[57] However, there is still nonspecificity involved with using this approach, and again, these growth factors only activate on aged skin cells (**Table 2**).

Although these 3 treatments have been considered for its role in decelerating skin aging, there are still disadvantages involved with their use. The most popular products are derived from the supernatant of cell cultures or the cytoplasmic contents of fetal epithelial cells. These products contain a great many biologically active substances and it is not known which contribute to the desired effect or even an undesired effect, such as tumorigenesis (**Fig. 5**A). Another drawback is the lack of standardization seen in what growth factors and proteins are being made and applied to.[39]

APPLICATIONS OF *LGR6+* STEM CELLS AND DEFENSINS

A new approach to aid in skin aging could be the use of defensins to activate *Lgr6+* stem cells (see **Table 1**). Unlike past treatments, defensins would only target *Lgr6+* cells, as opposed to many potential targets that may not only be helpful but also be deleterious or even tumorigenic in skin tissue (**Fig. 5**B); the investigators were not able to find any publications with respect to involvement of defensins into cancer-related pathways. Moreover, some tissues respond to tumor growth by enhanced expression of defensins as a natural protective immune response.[58,59] Studies also show the ability of defensins to suppress tumor growth both in vitro and in vivo.[59–62] In addition, *Lgr6+* cells are quiescent when compared with

Table 2
Generations in stem cell skin care

	1 Plant Stem Cells	2 Growth Factors from Conditioned Medium	3 Growth Factors (Defined)	4 Target-specific Stem Cell Activators
What Is This?	Plant Stem Cells	Growth Factors from Conditioned Medium	Growth Factors (Defined)	Target-specific Stem Cell Activators
Formulation	Undefined: mixture of active molecules	Undefined: mixture of growth factors—everything that cells release during in vitro culture	Defined: predefined composition of growth factors	Defined: predefined composition of natural peptides
Type of activation	Nonspecific: "switch-on of everything" mechanism Low efficacy	Nonspecific: "switch-on of everything" mechanism Contains TGF-β, potent cancer trigger	Nonspecific: "switch-on of everything"-mechanism	Highly specific: peptide (defensins) activate specific stem cells (*Lgr6+* stem cells)
What it does?	Forces "Old" and "exhausted" skin cells work even harder than before	Forces "Old" and "exhausted" skin cells work even harder than before	Forces "Old" and "exhausted" skin cells work even harder than before	Creates "New" and "fresh" skin cells using resource of our own body

A

GROWTH FACTORS
non-specific activation,
"switch-on of everything"-mechanism

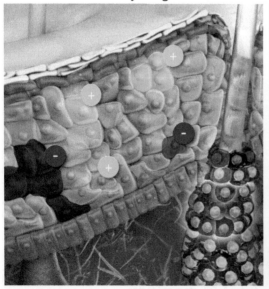

B

DEFENSINS
activation of specific cell type
to do specific job

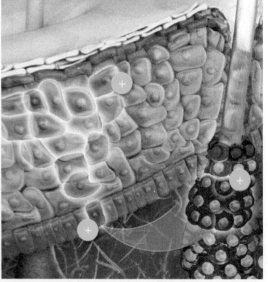

Fig. 5. Nonspecific versus specific targeting. (*A*) Because of the variety of functions, growth factors have an ability to activate and stimulate the different cells in skin including potentially "unstable" tumorigenic cells; therefore, the activation by growth factors is nonspecific and is based on a "switch-on of everything" mechanism. (*B*) Defensins activate only 1 specific cell type in skin, *Lgr6+* stem cells, thus representing a target-specific activation.

basal stem cells and reside in the isthmus, which is not as directly exposed to UV radiation, thus *Lgr6+* cells would have accumulated less mutations and damage than basal stem cells.[18] Thus, by activating these cells, there would be differentiation and proliferation of less damaged keratinocytes.

In a 6-week pilot study,[63] it was observed that there was a global improvement in wrinkle reduction and decreased skin oil production in the 22 subjects who used synthetic α-defensin 5– and β-defensin 3–based skin care regimen. To affirm these findings, a placebo-controlled, double-blind study across multiple medical centers was carried out with 45 subjects for 12 weeks. The results of this study followed those from the pilot, suggesting some potential for the use of defensins as a skin therapy.

In a randomized, double-blind, placebo multicenter controlled study of 45 patients, the same defensin-based 3-product skin care regimen was shown to be effective for global signs of skin aging on the face and neck.[64] The full formula regimen caused a significant ($P = .027$) increased thickness of the epidermis as seen in histology, not seen in the placebo group, with no signs of inflammation (**Fig. 6**). No excessive cell proliferation was detected in either group as measured by Ki67-immunohistochemistry. Reduction in visible pores, superficial wrinkles, oiliness, pigmentation, and improvement of skin evenness were statistically significant (**Fig. 7**). A trend for improvement was also observed in skin elasticity, transepidermal water loss, and hydration; these did not achieve statistical significance. Ultrasound and histopathology demonstrated increases in dermal thickness in individual patients, without statistical significance (**Fig. 8**). Comprehensive improvement in all 5 parameters, including visible pores, hyperpigmentation, superficial and deep wrinkles, and epidermal thickness, was statistically significant when the subset of participants assigned for histology in full formula group was compared with the placebo group participants.

Although further investigation must be done to fully understand the mechanisms behind defensins and skin repair, this therapy provides a new avenue for a more targeted treatment in skin aging.

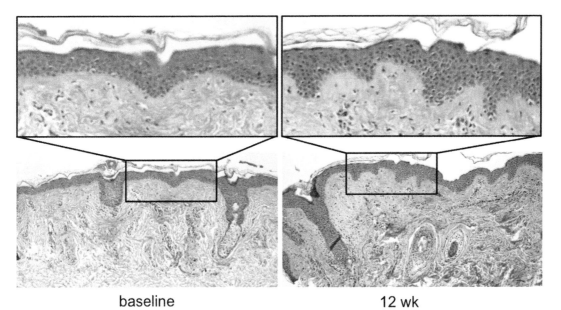

baseline   12 wk

Fig. 6. The defensin-based full formula causes thickening of the epidermis and dermis without visible signs of inflammation. Hematoxylin and eosin staining of skin biopsy samples collected from participants of the full formula group. The images indicate an increased number of keratinocytes in the epidermis and the thickening of the epidermis, observed in all participants of the full formula group assigned for histopathologic evaluation. Photos were taken at 10x magnification. (*From* Taub A, Bucay V, Keller G, et al. Multi-center, double-blind, vehicle-controlled clinical trial of an alpha and beta defensin-containing anti-aging skin care regimen with clinical, histopathologic, immunohistochemical, photographic, and ultrasound evaluation. J Drugs Dermatol 2018;17(4):426–41; with permission.)

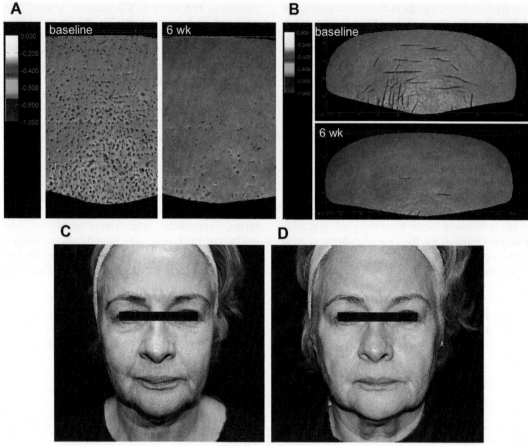

Fig. 7. Comprehensive improvement of the signs of skin aging with the defensin-based full formula. (*A*) Three-dimensional (3D) images of patient's skin (forehead) demonstrating the reduction of visible pores. The deepest areas of pores are shown in blue; the low-profile pores are shown in red-yellow. (*B*) 3D images of participant's skin (forehead). The deepest areas of wrinkles are shown in blue; the low-profile wrinkles are shown in red-yellow. (*C, D*) High-resolution photograph of a participant in the full formula group at baseline (*C*) and after 12 weeks (*D*). (*From [A, B]* Taub A, Bucay V, Keller G, et al. Multi-center, double-blind, vehicle-controlled clinical trial of an alpha and beta defensin-containing anti-aging skin care regimen with clinical, histopathologic, immunohistochemical, photographic, and ultrasound evaluation. J Drugs Dermatol 2018;17(4):426–41; with permission.)

SUMMARY

Currently, different skin therapies are emerging to treat and reverse the signs of aging. One approach is the utilization of growth factors to activate cell populations in the skin.[39] Initially starting with plant stem cells, to conditioned medium growth factors, and finally to defined growth factors, there is increasing specificity in the growth factors being applied but there are several disadvantages to these 3 treatments. First is the lack of specificity to target cells such that these stem cells and growth factors can activate cells that are not normally involved in skin rejuvenation and be deleterious or tumorigenic. In addition, there are concerns with the efficacy and safety of these treatments as the composition of growth factors are not fully defined

and there is a dearth of clinical research to affirm how effective these treatments are. Another aspect to their disadvantage is that all 3 activate aged basal stem cells that have accumulated photodamage, genetic mutations, and epigenetic alterations. By activating these cells, the differentiated keratinocytes will still possess these damages, thus not decelerating aging at an optimal rate.

Nevertheless, new findings demonstrate that certain stem cell populations in the hair follicle can facilitate in wound healing by creating long-term keratinocyte progenitors as well as appendages such as the hair follicle and sebaceous gland. One population of note is *Lgr6*+stem cell located in the hair follicle isthmus. This multipotent stem cells act as skin's master stem cells and in cases where there is wounding or other insults, these

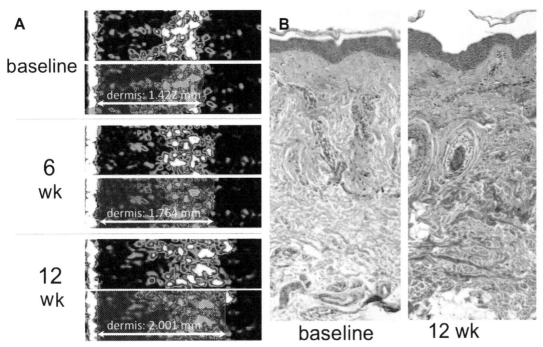

Fig. 8. Participants of the defensin-based full formula group demonstrated increase in dermal thickness. (A) High-resolution skin ultrasound demonstrates the increase in dermal thickness in the best participant. Dermis area is highlighted in red. Original US image is shown above the red-highlighted image. (B) Hematoxylin and eosin staining of skin biopsy samples showing increased dermal thickness. Photos were taken at 10x magnification. (From Taub A, Bucay V, Keller G, et al. Multi-center, double-blind, vehicle-controlled clinical trial of an alpha and beta defensin-containing anti-aging skin care regimen with clinical, histopathologic, immunohistochemical, photographic, and ultrasound evaluation. J Drugs Dermatol 2018;17(4):426–41; with permission.)

cells can proliferate and reprogram to epidermal fates and create new basal stem cells and, eventually, new keratinocytes.[33] In order for Lgr6+ cells to migrate into the wound bed, defensins must be present to target and activate these cells. β-defensin peptides are produced by the skin in cases where innate immunity is needed. Not only does it have immunomodulatory qualities but it also can specifically act on Lgr6+ cells for migration and proliferation onto the wound bed.[33]

Using this mechanism, further applications can be done in terms of skin aging therapy. Synthetic B-defensin 3 or A-defensin 5 has some advantages over previous growth factor treatments.[33] Each application will have a known composition because only defensins and a vehicle are necessary. Because defensins specifically target Lgr6+ cells, there will not be issues of inappropriate activation of other cell types. This approach would also activate a stem cell population that can produce basal stem cells and keratinocytes with less genetic damage and more signaling responsiveness in comparison to the keratinocytes that were derived from aged basal cells. Pilot studies have demonstrated that a composition of

defensins, topically applied on intact skin, dramatically improve overall quality of epidermis and comprehensively address the visible signs of aging skin. The observing effect may be caused by defensin-activated repopulation of epidermis with new and "healthy" basal cells following the increase of epidermal mass. Normalized/refreshed epidermis may enhance the performance of dermis renewal and function.

REFERENCES

1. Till JE, Mcculloch EA. A direct measurement of the radiation sensitivity of normal mouse bone marrow cells. Radiat Res 1961;14:213–22.
2. Thomas E, Storb R, Clift RA, et al. Bone-marrow transplantation (first of two parts). N Engl J Med 1975;292(16):832–43.
3. Schulz TC. Concise review: manufacturing of pancreatic endoderm cells for clinical trials in type 1 diabetes. Stem Cells Transl Med 2015;4(8): 927–31.
4. ClinicalTrials.gov. A safety, tolerability, and efficacystudy of VC-01™ combination product in subjects with type I diabetes mellitus. Available

at: https://clinicaltrials.gov/ct2/show/NCT02239354. Accessed April 14, 2017.

5. ClinicalTrials.gov. Safety of a single, intravitreal injection of human retinal progenitor cells (jCell) in retinitis pigmentosa. Available at: https://clinicaltrials.gov/ct2/show/NCT02320812. Accessed April 14, 2017.

6. ClinicalTrials.gov. Safety study of GRNOPC1 in spinal cord injury. Available at: https://clinicaltrials.gov/ct2/show/NCT01217008. Accessed April 14, 2017.

7. Lopez-Otin C, Blasco MA, Partridge L, et al. The hallmarks of aging. Cell 2013;153(6):1194–217.

8. Lee AS, Tang C, Rao MS, et al. Tumorigenicity as a clinical hurdle for pluripotent stem cell therapies. Nat Med 2013;19(8):998–1004.

9. Peterson SE, Garitaonandia I, Loring JF. The tumorigenic potential of pluripotent stem cells: what can we do to minimize it? Bioessays 2016;38(Suppl 1): S86–95.

10. King NM, Perrin J. Ethical issues in stem cell research and therapy. Stem Cell Res Ther 2014; 5(4):85.

11. Yoshihara M, Hayashizaki Y, Murakawa Y. Genomic instability of iPSCs: challenges towards their clinical applications. Stem Cell Rev 2017;13(1):7–16.

12. Hass R, Kasper C, Böhm S, et al. Different populations and sources of human mesenchymal stem cells (MSC): a comparison of adult and neonatal tissue-derived MSC. Cell Commun Signal 2011;9:12.

13. Zha Y, Masiello D, McMillan M, et al. CBP/catenin antagonist safely eliminates drug-resistant leukemia-initiation cells. Oncogene 2016;35(28):3705–17.

14. Plikus MV, Gay DL, Treffeisen E, et al. Epithelial stem cells and implications for wound repair. Semin Cell Dev Biol 2012;23:946–53.

15. Ito M, Liu Y, Yang Z, et al. Stem cells in the hair follicle bulge contribute to wound repair but not to homeostasis of the epidermis. Nat Med 2005; 11(12):1351–4.

16. Gordon W, Andersen B. A nervous hedgehog rolls into the hair follicle stem cell scene. Cell Stem Cell 2011;8:459–60.

17. Snippert HJ, Haegebarth A, Kasper M, et al. Lgr6 marks stem cells in the hair follicle that generate all cell lineages of the skin. Science 2010;327: 1385–9.

18. Campisi J, d'Adda di Fagagna F. Cellular senescence: when bad things happen to good cells. Nat Rev Mol Cell Biol 2007;8(9):729–40.

19. Potten CS, Bullock JC. Cell kinetic studies in the epidermis of the mouse: I. Changes in labeling index with time after tritiated thymidine administration. Experientia 1983;39:1125–9.

20. Clayton E, Doupe DP, Klein AM, et al. A single type of progenitor cell maintains normal epidermis. Nature 2007;446:185–9.

21. Doupe DP, Jones PH. Interfollicular epidermal homeostasis: a response to Gradually, '25 years of epidermal stem cell research'. J Invest Dermatol 2012;132:2096–7.

22. Jaks V, Barker N, Kasper M, et al. Lgr5 marks cycling, yet long-lived, hair follicle stem cells. Nat Genet 2008;40:1291–9.

23. Vidal VP, Chaboissier MC, Lutzkendorf S, et al. Sox9 is essential for outer root sheath differentiation and the formation of the hair stem cell compartment. Curr Biol 2005;15(15):1340–51.

24. Fuchs E. Skin stem cells: rising to the surface. J Cell Biol 2008;180(2):273–84.

25. Ito M, Yang Z, Andl T, et al. Wnt-dependent de novo hair follicle regeneration in adult mouse skin after wounding. Nature 2007;447:316–20.

26. Levy V, Lindon C, Zheng Y, et al. Epidermal stem cells arise from the hair follicle after wounding. FASEB J 2007;21:1358.

27. Cotsarelis G, Sun TT, Lavker RM. Label-retaining cells reside in the bulge area of the pilosebaceous unit: implications for follicular stem cells, hair cycle, and skin carcinogenesis. Cell 1990;61:1329–37.

28. Nowak JA, Polak L, Paroli AH, et al. Hair follicle stem cells are specified and function in early skin morphogenesis. Cell Stem Cell 2008;3(1):33–43.

29. Jensen KB, Collins CA, Nascimento E, et al. Lrig1 expression defines a distinct multipotent stem cell population in mammalian epidermis. Cell Stem Cell 2009;4(5):427–39.

30. Jaks V, Kasper M, Toftgard R. The hair follicle-a stem cell zoo. Exp Cell Res 2010;316(8):1422–8.

31. Horsley V, O'Carrol D, Tooze R, et al. Blimp1 defines a progenitor population that governs cellular input to the sebaceous gland. Cell 2006;126(3):597–609.

32. Blanpain C. Skin regeneration and repair. Nature 2010;464:686–7.

33. Lough D, Dai H, Yang M, et al. Stimulation of the follicular bulge LGR5+ and LGR6+ stem cells with the gut-derived human alpha defensin 5 results in decreased bacterial presence, enhanced wound healing, and hair growth from tissues devoid of adnexal structures. Plast Reconstr Surg 2013; 132(5):1159–71.

34. Lough DM, Yang M, Blum A, et al. Transplantation of the LGR6+ epithelial stem cell into full-thickness cutaneous wounds results in enhanced healing, nascent hair follicle development, and augmentation of angiogenic analystes. Plast Reconstr Surg 2014; 133(3):579–90.

35. Zasloff M. Antimicrobial peptides in health and disease. N Engl J Med 2002;347:1199–200.

36. Kiatsurayanon C, Niyonsaba F, Smithrithee R, et al. Host defense (antimicrobial) peptide, human β-defensin-3, improves the function of the epithelial tight-junction barrier in human keratinocytes. J Invest Dermatol 2014;134(8):2163–73.

37. Quan T, He T, Kang S, et al. Solar ultraviolet irradiation reduces collagen in photoaged human skin by blocking transforming growth factor-β type II receptor/Smad signaling. Am J Pathol 2004;165(3): 741–51.

38. Yamamoto Y, Gaynor RB. Therapeutic potential of inhibition of the NF-kappaB pathway in the treatment of inflammation and cancer. J Clin Invest 2001; 107(2):135–42.

39. Fabi S, Sundaram H. The potential of topical and injectable growth factors and cytokines for skin rejuvenation. Facial Plast Surg 2014;30:157–71.

40. Beanes SR, Dang C, Soo C, et al. Down-regulation of decorin, a transforming growth factor-β modulator, is associated with scarless fetal wound healing. J Pediatr 2001;36(11):1666–71.

41. Hu MSM, Rennet RC, McArdle A, et al. The role of stem cells during scarless skin wound healing. Adv Wound Care 2014;3(4):304–14.

42. Malek A, Bersinger NA. Human placental stem cells: biomedical potential and clinical relevance. J Stem Cells 2011;6:75–92.

43. Mehta RC, Fitzpatrick RE. Endogenous growth factors as cosmeceuticals. Dermatol Ther 2007;20(5): 350–9.

44. Sundaram H, Mehta RC, Norine JA. Topically applied physiologically balanced growth factors: a new paradigm of skin rejuvenation. J Drugs Dermatol 2009;8(5):4–13.

45. Moulin V. Growth factors in skin wound healing. Eur J Cell Biol 1995;68(1):1–7.

46. Cheng M, Wang H, Yoshida R, et al. Platelets and plasma proteins are both required to stimulate collagen gene expression by anterior cruciate ligament cells in three-dimensional culture. Tissue Eng Part A 2010;16(5):1479–89.

47. Wu JJ, Weinstein GD, Kricorian GJ, et al. Topical kinetin 0.1% lotion for improving the signs and symptoms of rosacea. Clin Exp Dermatol 2007; 32(6):693–5.

48. Dermatology Times. Behind the hype in stem cell therapy. Available at: http://dermatologytimes. modernmedicine.com/dermatology-times/news/ dermatology-experts-set-stem-cell-record-straight. Accessed April 14, 2017.

49. Fitzpatrick RE, Rostan EF. Reversal of photodamage with topical growth factors: a pilot study. J Cosmet Laser Ther 2003;5(1):25–34.

50. Meirelles Lda S, Fontes AM, Covas DT, et al. Mechanisms involved in the therapeutic properties of mesenchymal stem cells. Cytokine Growth Factor Rev 2009;20(5–6):419–27.

51. Falanga V, Su Wen Qian V, Danielpour D, et al. Hypoxia upregulates the synthesis of TGF-β by human dermal fibroblasts. J Invest Dermatol 1991;97(4): 634–7.

52. de Gramont A, Faivre S, Raymond E. Novel TGF-β inhibitors ready for prime time in onco-immunology. Oncoimmunology 2016;6(1):e1257453.

53. Neuzillet C, Tijeras-Raballand A, Cohen R, et al. Targeting the TGFβ pathway for cancer therapy. Pharmacol Ther 2015;147:22–31.

54. Lopez-Novoa JM, Nieto MA. Inflammation and EMT: an alliance towards organ fibrosis and cancer progression. EMBO Mol Med 2009;1:303–14.

55. Jakowlew SB. Transforming growth factor-beta in cancer and metastasis. Cancer Metastasis Rev 2006;25:435–57.

56. Thisse B, Thisse C. Functions and regulations of fibroblast growth factor signaling during embryonic development. Dev Biol 2005;287(2):390–402.

57. Dreher F. A novel matrikine-like micro-protein complex (MPC) technology for topical skin rejuvenation. J Drugs Dermatol 2016;15(4):457–64.

58. Semple F, Dorin JR. β-Defensins: multifunctional modulators of infection, inflammation and more? J Innate Immun 2012;4(4):337–48.

59. Hanaoka Y, Yamaguchi Y, Yamamoto H, et al. In vitro and in vivo anticancer activity of human β-defensin-3 and its mouse homolog. Anticancer Res 2016; 36(11):5999–6004.

60. Lichtenstein A, Ganz T, Selested ME, et al. In vitro tumor cell cytolysis mediated by peptide defensins of human and rabbit granulocytes. Blood 1986;68: 1407–10.

61. Biragy A, Ruffini PA, Leifer CA, et al. Toll-like receptor 4-dependent activation of dendritic cells by β-defensin 2. Science 2002;298:1025–9.

62. Biragy A, Surenhu M, Yang D, et al. Mediators of innate immunity that target immature, but not mature, dendritic cells induce antitumor immunity when genetically fused with nonimmunogenic tumor antigens. J Immunol 2001;167:6644–53.

63. Keller G. The Advanced Aesthetics & Cosmetic Dermatology Symposium 2017. Keller G. Stem cell stimulation and skin rejuvenation: current practices. Available at: http://aacdmeeting.org/overview/. Accessed April 14, 2017.

64. Taub A, Bucay V, Keller G, et al. Multi-Center, Double-Blind, Vehicle-Controlled Clinical Trial of an Alpha and Beta Defensin-Containing Anti-Aging Skin Care Regimen With Clinical, Histopathologic, Immunohistochemical, Photographic, and Ultrasound Evaluation. J Drugs Dermatol 2018;17(4): 426–41.

Platelet-Rich Plasma for Skin Rejuvenation and Tissue Fill

Jiahui Lin, MD, Anthony P. Sclafani, MD*

KEYWORDS

- Platelet-rich plasma • Platelet-rich fibrin matrix • Skin rejuvenation • Tissue fill • Autologous fat graft
- Laser resurfacing

KEY POINTS

- Platelet preparations, including platelet-rich plasma (PRP) and platelet-rich fibrin matrix (PRFM), contain high concentrations of growth factors that facilitate wound healing.
- Platelet preparations are generally safe to use, as they are derived from patients' own blood and, thus, are typically inexpensive to obtain.
- Platelet preparations have been used alone for small-volume tissue fill, such as for treatment of facial wrinkles, to help maintain contour when performing autologous fat grafts and to improve cosmetic outcomes and decrease recovery time after laser resurfacing.
- PRFM may be a better option compared with PRP, because of its slower release of growth factors and its greater similarity to the natural clotting and wound healing process.
- More robust studies are necessary to definitively characterize the benefits of platelet preparations for facial rejuvenation and tissue fill.

INTRODUCTION

Platelet-rich plasma (PRP) has been one of various platelet preparations that have been used for wound healing, facial rejuvenation, and recovery after surgery. Although platelet preparations use is well documented in orthopedic and dental surgery, they have not yet been widely adopted in facial plastic surgery. Platelet preparations contain growth factors that enhance the production of collagen and fibronectin, promote angiogenesis, and improve wound healing.[1] Although studies abound, there are few robust randomized controlled trials. Most published literature consists of case reports or small case series. The preparation and specific type of platelet preparation used are also not always specified, making comparisons and further studies difficult. Additionally, objective outcomes are difficult to measure and not always reported, thereby limiting the results of many published studies. This article focuses specifically on the available data on the use of platelet preparations in facial skin rejuvenation and tissue fill.

WHAT IS PLATELET-RICH PLASMA?

All platelet preparations start with autologous whole blood, from which platelets and other cells and proteins can be harvested (Table 1). Various types of platelet preparations exist and are classified based on their concentrations of leukocytes and fibrin polymerization as a result of the preparation technique.[2] All techniques involve blood collection immediately before use and one or more centrifugation steps. At a minimum, centrifugation separates a red blood cell (RBC) layer from a supernatant platelet-poor plasma (PPP) layer

Department of Otolaryngology–Head and Neck Surgery, Weill Cornell Medicine, 1305 York Avenue, Fifth Floor, New York, NY 10021, USA
* Corresponding author. Department of Otolaryngology–Head and Neck Surgery, Weill Greenberg Center, Weill Cornell Medicine, 1305 York Avenue, Fifth Floor, New York, NY 10021.
E-mail address: ans9243@med.cornell.edu

Facial Plast Surg Clin N Am 26 (2018) 439–446
https://doi.org/10.1016/j.fsc.2018.06.005
1064-7406/18/© 2018 Elsevier Inc. All rights reserved.

Table 1
Types of platelet preparations and their properties

	Leukocyte Poor	Leukocyte Rich
PRP	P-PRP (small volume, weak/minimal fibrin polymerization)	L-PRP (significant WBCs, small volume, weak/minimal fibrin polymerization)
PRF	P-PRF/PRFM (larger volume, strong/dense fibrin polymerization)	L-PRF (significant WBCs, larger volume, strong/dense fibrin polymerization)

Abbreviations: L-PRF, leukocyte-poor platelet-rich fibrin; L-PRP, leukocyte-rich PRP; P-PRF, leukocyte-poor platelet-rich fibrin; PRF, platelet-rich fibrin; PRFM, platelet-rich fibrin matrix; P-PRP, leukocyte-poor PRF; WBCs, white blood cells.

Adapted from Dohan Ehrenfest DM, Rasmusson L, Albrektsson T. Classification of platelet concentrates: from pure platelet-rich plasma (P-PRP) to leucocyte- and platelet-rich fibrin (L-PRF). Trends Biotechnol 2009;27:165; with permission.

and a buffy coat layer in between that is rich in platelets and leukocytes. Additional centrifugation of the supernatant and buffy coat layers can yield 2 types of PRP: leukocyte-poor (or pure) PRP (P-PRP; leukocytes are separated from the platelets, which are subsequently concentrated in a small volume of plasma) and leukocyte-rich PRP (L-PRP; platelets and leukocytes together are concentrated in a small volume of plasma).

Both types of PRP typically require an activation step to release the growth factors with calcium chloride and/or thrombin. P-PRP was the first form of platelet concentrate developed for topical use. However, it required the support of a transfusion laboratory or cell separator in order to process out the leukocytes. Protocols that did not rely on such systems were often inconsistent and would yield L-PRP instead. Thus, L-PRP was developed, initially as a means to create PRP without a cell separator and later to purposefully include leukocytes for their anti-infectious and immune regulatory effects. Furthermore, leukocytes are known to produce large amounts of vascular endothelial growth factor (VEGF), which could further promote angiogenesis.[3,4]

Platelet-rich fibrin matrix (PRFM) differs from PRP, as it is larger in volume, has a lower platelet concentration, and includes fibrin that develops into a 3-dimensional matrix to bind growth factors and cells.[5] The most common commercially available form is leukocyte-poor platelet-rich fibrin (PRF) (sometimes referred to PRFM or P-PRF), in which collected blood is centrifuged at a low speed without anticoagulants in the presence of a thixotropic separator gel to produce 3 layers: a layer below the gel containing the RBCs and most white blood cells (WBCs), a buffy coat of platelets on the upper surface of the gel, and a supernatant PPP layer, which has a fibrinogen content equivalent to that of normal plasma. The plasma and buffy coat are then removed and used together. Activation with calcium, thrombin, or even through direct contact with tissue leads to conversion of fibrinogen to a polymerized fibrin, platelet degranulation, and release of growth factors from alpha granules. The fibrin network formed provides sites for binding and localization of growth factors and is also theorized to provide a scaffold for cellular migration and collagen deposition. It is thought that this preparation mimics natural clot formation and the wound response more closely.

A leukocyte-rich PRF (L-PRF) preparation also exists, but it has not widely been used for facial plastic surgical applications. The technique is similar to PRP methods with a few exceptions. After the first centrifugation, the buffy coat and PPP are transferred into a calcium chloride tube. A P-PRF clot can be formed after the second centrifugation and subsequently applied.

PRP is the most common commercially available platelet preparation. It classically contains 4 to 7 times the amount of platelets compared with the patients' baseline.[6] Its clinical benefits are largely attributed to the growth factors that are contained within alpha granules, including platelet-derived growth factor, epithelial growth factor, and VEGF.[7,8] These granules also contain other factors that may modulate inflammation and increase membrane permeability, including serotonin, histamine, dopamine, and adenosine.[9] Once the platelet preparation is activated, typically by calcium chloride or thrombin, these growth factors and bioactive factors are released from the alpha granules to act locally where the PRP is applied. When applied, PRP has been postulated to increase dermal fibroblast proliferation, increase the expression of matrix metalloproteinases (from leukocytes) to remove photodamaged extracellular matrix, augment the production of collagen, and promote wound healing via increased expression of G1 cell cycle regulators.[10,11]

It is important to distinguish between these different types of platelet preparations and reported preparation techniques. Although they are clearly delineated here, it is not always obvious in published reports, as most preparations are commonly referred to simply as *PRP*. In the review to follow, the type or platelet preparation is specified (if stated or if it can be determined based on the published methodology; if unable to be determined, it will be referred to as a platelet preparation).

Commercially Available Platelet Preparation Systems

As mentioned earlier, several different systems are commercially available for isolating useable platelet preparations. The authors advocate no one system over another, and the links to manufacturers' proprietary resources are provided in this section to facilitate the reader's evaluation. All of the following devices work with a tabletop centrifuge, although some have larger centrifuges to be used in a hospital setting for larger volumes. The Harvest SmartPrep System (Terumo BCT, Inc, Lakewood, CO) works on a system of sequential centrifugation with a free-floating barrier to produce a platelet concentrate (L-PRP). Disposables are available to produce 3 to 4 or 8 to 10 mL of L-PRP using 30 or 60 mL of peripheral blood, respectively (https://www.harvesttech.com/clinician/clinician-home/prp/products). The MagellanPRP device (Isto Biologics, St Louis, MO) uses a disposable separation chamber that relies on dual-speed centrifugation to produce L-PRPs of customizable platelet concentrations (6–12 × over peripheral blood) and volumes. It requires 30 to 60 mL of blood to produce 10 to 30 mL of PRP (http://www.arteriocyte.com/magellanprptrade.html). The Arthrex Angel system (Arthrex, Inc, Naples, FL) relies on centrifugation to separate PPP from the platelet fraction and the RBC fraction and sensors to isolate these 3 streams based on the platelet absorption of 470 nm light and RBC absorption of 940 nm light. It requires 40 to 180 mL of peripheral blood and produces a variable volume of PRP, as the concentrations of platelets and WBCs can be programmed. This system can produce an L-PRP with up to 18 times the platelet concentration seen in peripheral blood (https://www.arthrex.com/orthobiologics/arthrex-angel-system/resources). The Arthrex ACP system will produce approximately 5 to 10 mL of L-PRF from as little as 15 mL of blood. Blood is centrifuged in a disposable double syringe, allowing harvest of plasma and the buffy coat after centrifugation (https://www.arthrex.com/orthobiologics/autologous-conditioned-plasma). The Biomet GPS III system (Biomet Biologics, Warsaw, IN) relies on centrifugation of a disposable separation chamber with a fixed buoy system to produce an L-PRP and requires 27 to 54 mL of whole blood to produce 3 to 6 mL of PRP (http://www.biomet.com/wps/wcm/connect/internet/495a2ac6-b2ed-48ec-930b-0cd0bb41ed0c/BBI0022.0_081508.pdf?MOD=AJPERES). The GenesisCS Pure PRP system (Accellerated Biologics, Tequesta, FL) uses 2 separate disposable separation chambers and double centrifugation to produce a P-PRP or, if desired, an L-PRP containing RBCs. Thirty to 120 mL of blood can be processed to yield 3 to 12 mL of PRP (https://nebula.wsimg.com/c13f34a00ca295a489375294dcd23cef?AccessKeyId=54D857698A1C97A5D719&disposition=0&alloworigin=1). The GenesisCS PRP system (Accellerated Biologics, Tequesta, FL) uses disposables with maximum volumes of 30, 60, or 120 mL (adjustable in increments of 10 mL) of blood to produce up to 3, 6, or 12 mL of L-PRP, respectively, by single-stage centrifugation, although the RBC content is higher than with other devices (https://nebula.wsimg.com/d92c6014e3a04904ad0d3bd4dd5d4eff?AccessKeyId=54D857698A1C97A5D719&disposition=0&alloworigin=1). Both the RegenKit THT (Stryker, Kalamazoo, MI) and the Selphyl (UBS Aesthetics, Bethlehem, PA) systems rely on a single centrifugation of a disposable vacuum tube with a thixotropic separator gel to isolate 4 to 5 mL of PRF from 8 to 9 mL of whole blood, with a 1- to 2-fold concentration of platelets. Both the RegenKit THT and Selphyl systems produce a P-PRF (https://www.regenlabusa.com/#regen™-products) and are the simplest to use.

In Vitro and In Vivo Studies

The wide variety of platelet preparation techniques is a testament to the desire to optimize the platelet concentration. As most of the growth factors are purported to be contained in the platelet-rich component, many studies focus on increasing the platelet concentration. Interestingly, an in vitro study on L-PRP and PPP suggested that these assumptions may not tell the entire story.[12] First, activation of L-PRP to increase proliferation of human adipose-derived stem cells and human dermal fibroblasts reached a maximum efficacy with a PRP concentration of 5%, but higher concentrations (of up to 20%) were less effective in stimulating cell growth. This finding provides some evidence that positive influence on cellular effects may be related to the ratio of growth factors and their sustained release, rather than pure concentration. Secondly, although activated L-PRP showed significantly increased cell proliferation compared with nonactivated L-PRP (as expected), activated PPP had a similar effect compared with its nonactivated counterpart, suggesting that the oft-discarded PPP may also provide some benefit to wound healing.

Various animal studies have been performed to characterize the benefits of platelet preparations as well. In one study, wrinkles were induced via ultraviolet B in mice.[13] Subcutaneous injections of L-PRP seemed to significantly improve skin roughness compared with placebo saline injections. Several animal studies have also shown some benefits to tissue fill using fat grafts. Injection of activated PRP mixed with fat grafts using the Coleman method into the scalps of nude mice significantly increased fat graft weight and volume, as well as vascularization, compared with a control group without PRP after 10 weeks.[14] Another study noted improved maintenance of fat grafts transplanted into rabbit ears with P-PRP enrichment compared with controls.[15] These investigators also found decreased necrosis and fibrosis as well as increased viable adipocytes and blood vessels in those transplanted with P-PRP. Only one study using L-PRP in mice showed no effect on fat graft survival, but it did not seem to use an extrinsic activation method.[16] In humans, deep dermal and subdermal injections of PRFM into the upper arms have resulted in increased activated fibroblasts, new collagen deposition, development of new blood vessels, intradermal collections of adipocytes, and stimulation of subdermal adipocytes on histologic review (**Fig. 1**).[17]

SMALL-VOLUME TISSUE FILL

Traditionally, tissue fillers have been used for various applications on the face, including age-induced wrinkles, atrophic acne scars, photodamaged skin, and depressed skin. Heavier or higher viscosity fillers, such as calcium hydroxylapatite, have often been used for subdermal and

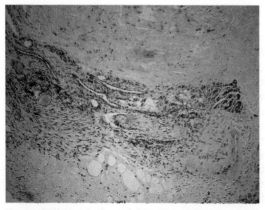

Fig. 1. Microscopic view of skin treated 19 days earlier with intradermal PRFM (hematoxylin-eosin stain, original magnification ×10).

subcutaneous injection.[18] Thinner fillers, such as monophasic hyaluronic acid (HA), are commonly used for dermal injections. Fat grafting provides more volume and is discussed separately.

In addition to injectable fillers, various studies have used topical application of growth factors to decrease wrinkles, improve the smoothness of skin, as well as improve wound healing after rejuvenating therapies.[19–22] There has been growing interest in using platelet preparations for facial rejuvenation and low-volume tissue fill, given their higher concentrations of autologous growth factors. Facial injections of platelet preparations have been shown to yield longer-term improvements with regard to skin turgor, smoothness, hydration, and overall vitality in a split-face study compared with injection of ready-made growth factors.[23] Most studies using platelet preparations in this manner have used them without the addition of other fillers.

Injections of PRP alone have showed mixed results. After injection of a platelet preparation in 20 women for improvement of facial wrinkles, a study found that at 8 weeks after treatment, the most significant improvements were in women less than 40 years old treated for nasolabial fold wrinkles.[24] In another study of 10 patients, 1.5 mL of L-PRP was intradermally injected in one session into the tear trough and crow's feet wrinkles bilaterally.[25] Although infraorbital color homogeneity improved significantly, there were no changes in wrinkle volume, melanin content, stratum corneum hydration, or visibility index. One study resulted in statistically significant improvement in skin firmness when a platelet preparation was applied to the forehead, malar area, and jaw using a dermaroller and injected into crow's feet wrinkles in 10 patients.[26] These treatments were applied 3 times at 2-week intervals. Yet another split-face study showed that injections of L-PRP in 20 patients into the upper infra-auricular area resulted in increased dermal collagen levels, compared with saline alone.[27] On the other hand, a study of 23 patients resulted in only 33% improvement in skin homogeneity and 30% in crow's feet wrinkles after monthly L-PRP injections for 3 months.[28] Only one study used P-PRP, which was injected intradermally in 10 patients and resulted in a significant increase in epidermal and papillary dermal thickness, collagen volume, and number of dermal fibroblasts.[29]

PRF has been postulated to yield better results than PRP, as it releases growth factors over a longer period of time. PRFM has been used to treat crow's feet wrinkles, tear troughs (**Fig. 2**), suborbital hollows, glabellar furrows, malar augmentation, zygomatic arch enhancement,

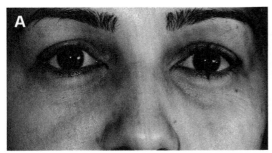
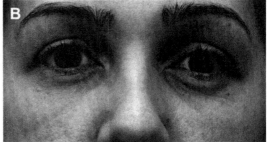

Fig. 2. (A) Pretreatment and (B) posttreatment close-up views of patient treated for tear trough deformity.

correction of nasolabial and marionette folds, and acne scars.[30] PRFM injection into the nasolabial folds (**Fig. 3**) in 15 patients showed improvements in the wrinkle assessment score by 12 weeks after treatment in 80% of patients.[5] Another study of subdermal PRFM injections in 16 patients into the nasolabial folds showed a significant increase in thickness and volume 3 months after treatment.[31] Yet another study of 12 patients undergoing 3 sessions of PRFM dermal injections into the nasolabial folds, forehead, and cheeks resulted in improved skin texture, gross elasticity, smoothness, barrier, and capacitance function.[32]

Few studies have combined platelet preparations with other tissue fillers. In one study, a combination of HA and platelet preparation injections was shown to improve facial skin elasticity 6 months after treatment.[33] A much larger study of 2005 patients resulted in a 97% satisfaction rate after receiving L-PRP and basic fibroblast growth factor (FGF) injections to treat nasolabial folds, marionette lines, nasojugal grooves, supraorbital grooves, midcheek grooves, forehead, temple, and glabellar depressions.[34] These investigators previously found that PRP alone was not sufficient to achieve significant improvement, which prompted them to combine it with FGF.

AUTOLOGOUS FAT GRAFTS

Platelet preparations have been combined with fat grafts to help promote volume maintenance and decrease facial scarring. Although fat grafts have been used since the 1890s, resorption has been a chronically described problem.[35,36] In this setting, platelet preparations may increase graft longevity and decrease the length of recovery by promoting wound healing, providing nutrient support, increasing angiogenesis, and enhancing the proliferation of preadipocytes and adipose-derived stem cells.[37]

In 22 patients undergoing minimal access cranial suspension facelift, fat grafting, and L-PRP injection into the fat graft plane, significant improvement in aesthetic outcome and recovery time was achieved compared with 17 patients who underwent the same procedure without L-PRP.[38] However, another report showed no benefit when P-PRP was added to adipose-derived stem cell–enriched fat grafts for facelift, compared with stromal vascular fraction–enriched fat or adipose-derived stem cells, and ultimately increased inflammation and other vascular changes.[39] A study of 32 women compared facial lipofilling with L-PRP or saline and found that the addition of L-PRP did not significantly improve skin elasticity, volume retention, or

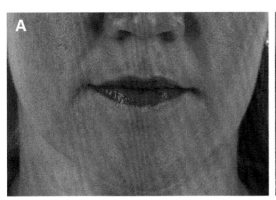
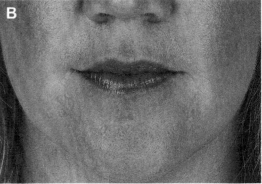

Fig. 3. (A) Pretreatment and (B) posttreatment close-up views of patient treated for deep nasolabial folds.

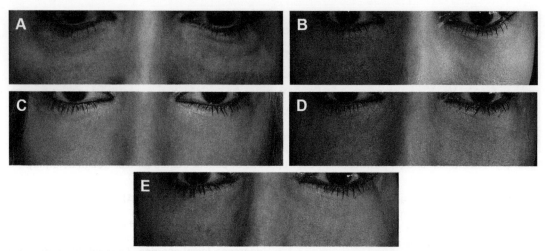

Fig. 4. Close-up images of patient before, during, and after serial treatment with PRFM. (*A*) Pretreatment; (*B*) 1 month after first treatment; (*C*) 6 months after first treatment; (*D*) 8 months after first, 2 months after second treatment; (*E*) 25, 6, and 4 months after first, second, and third treatments, respectively.

patient satisfaction.[40] However, it did significantly reduce recovery time after the procedure. Another study of 18 patients who underwent fat grafting with the Coleman technique and L-PRP injection also showed significantly reduced recovery time compared with 25 patients who underwent the procedure without L-PRP.[38]

Interestingly, because of the retention and slower release of growth factors from platelets with PRFM, there has been increasing interest in using this preparation over PRP for autologous fat grafts.[37] In 10 patients with facial burns or post-traumatic facial scars, PRFM admixed with autologous fat grafts was found to achieve maintenance of contour restoration after 1 year in 69% of patients, compared with only 39% in the control group of 10 patients treated with fat only.[41] Maintenance was measured by MRI and ultrasound imaging. Yet another study of 25 patients who received fat grafting with PRFM showed 70% contour maintenance volume after 1 year compared with 31% in the control group of 10 patients treated with only fat grafting.[42] However, a study of 49 patients with highly active antiretroviral therapy–associated lipoatrophy treated with autologous fat injection alone or with PRFM showed no significant differences between the two groups at 2 and 12 months posttreatment, evaluated by computed tomography imaging.[43]

LASER RESURFACING

Platelet preparations have also been combined with carbon dioxide (CO_2) fractional laser resurfacing techniques in order to augment the effects of the treatment as well as speed re-epithelization and wound healing after the procedure. In 14

patients with facial acne scarring, intradermal injection of L-PRP compared with saline injection on the contralateral side in conjunction with fractional CO_2 laser resurfacing showed a significantly shortened duration of postprocedure erythema, edema, and crusting as well as overall greater clinical improvement.[44] Another split-face study compared 15 patients intradermally injected with L-PRP on one side and saline on the other, in combination with a CO_2 fractional laser for acne scarring therapy.[45] After 3 treatments, 4 weeks apart, improvements were noted in skin smoothness with L-PRP treatment compared with saline as well as improved acne scar depth when measured by optical coherence tomography. Intradermal injection of L-PRP in combination with a CO_2 fractional laser was shown in yet another study to improve skin texture, elasticity, edema, erythema, and crusting using VISIA skin analysis compared with saline injections in 13 patients.[46] Yet another study showed improvements in the erythema index when L-PRP was applied with 1550-nm fractional erbium:glass laser facial resurfacing compared with no L-PRP, with increased dermal thickness in the L-PRP group histologically.[47]

CASE STUDY

A 36-year-old woman presented requesting improvement in the appearance of the area under and around her eyes. She stated that she did not want a significant recovery phase and had not been treated in the past, surgically or nonsurgically. The patient had evidence of moderate hollowing and skeletonization of her infraorbital rim as well as mild blepharochalasis (**Fig. 4**A). She was treated with PRFM injection after rejecting treatment with a low-density HA derivative. Good improvement was noted at the 1-month follow-up visit (**Fig. 4**B). She returned 6 months after the initial treatment noting some recurrence of hollowing (**Fig. 4**C) and was retreated with PRFM. Two months later, the hollowing was improved, but she now desired additional treatment in the naso-jugal trough (**Fig. 4**D). The patient has since noted stable improvement with good correction of the cosmetic deformity 25 months after the initial treatment (**Fig. 4**E).

SUMMARY

Platelet preparations are a safe and relatively inexpensive adjunctive therapy. Its high concentrations of growth factors may improve wound healing, recovery time, and cosmetic outcomes for facial rejuvenation. PRFM is in general a less expensive technique; it may also be more efficacious compared with PRP, given its slower release of growth factors and greater similarity to the natural clotting process. As an autologous material, platelet preparations generally have limited adverse tissue reactions and are an attractive option in facial rejuvenation. As a biological stimulant, appropriate expectations of the rapidity and degree of tissue volumizing are necessary. Given the current literature, more robust studies are necessary in order to validate these benefits.

REFERENCES

1. Sclafani AP, Romo T 3rd, Ukrainsky G, et al. Modulation of wound response and soft tissue ingrowth in synthetic and allogeneic implants with platelet concentrate. Arch Facial Plast Surg 2005;7:163–9.
2. Dohan Ehrenfest DM, Rasmusson L, Albrektsson T. Classification of platelet concentrates: from pure platelet-rich plasma (P-PRP) to leucocyte- and platelet-rich fibrin (L-PRF). Trends Biotechnol 2009;27:158–67.
3. El-Sharkawy H, Kantarci A, Deady J, et al. Platelet-rich plasma: growth factors and pro- and anti-inflammatory properties. J Periodontol 2007;78:661–9.
4. Werther K, Christensen IJ, Nielsen HJ. Determination of vascular endothelial growth factor (VEGF) in circulating blood: significance of VEGF in various leucocytes and platelets. Scand J Clin Lab Invest 2002;62:343–50.
5. Sclafani AP. Platelet-rich fibrin matrix for improvement of deep nasolabial folds. J Cosmet Dermatol 2010;9:66–71.
6. Marx RE. Platelet-rich plasma (PRP): what is PRP and what is not PRP? Implant Dent 2001;10:225–8.
7. Lubkowska A, Dolegowska B, Banfi G. Growth factor content in PRP and their applicability in medicine. J Biol Regul Homeost Agents 2012;26:3S–22S.
8. Marx RE. Platelet-rich plasma: evidence to support its use. J Oral Maxillofac Surg 2004;62:489–96.
9. Foster TE, Puskas BL, Mandelbaum BR, et al. Platelet-rich plasma: from basic science to clinical applications. Am J Sports Med 2009;37:2259–72.
10. Cho JW, Kim SA, Lee KS. Platelet-rich plasma induces increased expression of G1 cell cycle regulators, type I collagen, and matrix metalloproteinase-1 in human skin fibroblasts. Int J Mol Med 2012;29:32–6.
11. Kim DH, Je YJ, Kim CD, et al. Can platelet-rich plasma be used for skin rejuvenation? Evaluation of effects of platelet-rich plasma on human dermal fibroblast. Ann Dermatol 2011;23:424–31.
12. Kakudo N, Minakata T, Mitsui T, et al. Proliferation-promoting effect of platelet-rich plasma on human adipose-derived stem cells and human dermal fibroblasts. Plast Reconstr Surg 2008;122:1352–60.
13. Cho JM, Lee YH, Baek RM, et al. Effect of platelet-rich plasma on ultraviolet b-induced skin wrinkles in nude mice. J Plast Reconstr Aesthet Surg 2011;64:e31–9.
14. Oh DS, Cheon YW, Jeon YR, et al. Activated platelet-rich plasma improves fat graft survival in nude mice: a pilot study. Dermatol Surg 2011;37:619–25.
15. Pires Fraga MF, Nishio RT, Ishikawa RS, et al. Increased survival of free fat grafts with platelet-rich plasma in rabbits. J Plast Reconstr Aesthet Surg 2010;63:e818–22.
16. Por YC, Yeow VK, Louri N, et al. Platelet-rich plasma has no effect on increasing free fat graft survival in the nude mouse. J Plast Reconstr Aesthet Surg 2009;62:1030–4.
17. Sclafani AP, McCormick SA. Induction of dermal collagenesis, angiogenesis, and adipogenesis in human skin by injection of platelet-rich fibrin matrix. Arch Facial Plast Surg 2012;14:132–6.
18. Bass LS. Injectable filler techniques for facial rejuvenation, volumization, and augmentation. Facial Plast Surg Clin North Am 2015;23:479–88.
19. Fitzpatrick RE, Rostan EF. Reversal of photodamage with topical growth factors: a pilot study. J Cosmet Laser Ther 2003;5:25–34.
20. Atkin DH, Trookman NS, Rizer RL, et al. Combination of physiologically balanced growth factors with antioxidants for reversal of facial photodamage. J Cosmet Laser Ther 2010;12:14–20.
21. Mehta RC, Smith SR, Grove GL, et al. Reduction in facial photodamage by a topical growth factor product. J Drugs Dermatol 2008;7:864–71.
22. Fabi S, Sundaram H. The potential of topical and injectable growth factors and cytokines for skin rejuvenation. Facial Plast Surg 2014;30:157–71.

23. Gawdat HI, Tawdy AM, Hegazy RA, et al. Autologous platelet-rich plasma versus readymade growth factors in skin rejuvenation: a split face study. J Cosmet Dermatol 2017;16(2):258–64.

24. Elnehrawy NY, Ibrahim ZA, Eltoukhy AM, et al. Assessment of the efficacy and safety of single platelet-rich plasma injection on different types and grades of facial wrinkles. J Cosmet Dermatol 2017; 16:103–11.

25. Mehryan P, Zartab H, Rajabi A, et al. Assessment of efficacy of platelet-rich plasma (PRP) on infraorbital dark circles and crow's feet wrinkles. J Cosmet Dermatol 2014;13:72–8.

26. Yuksel EP, Sahin G, Aydin F, et al. Evaluation of effects of platelet-rich plasma on human facial skin. J Cosmet Laser Ther 2014;16:206–8.

27. Abuaf OK, Yildiz H, Baloglu H, et al. Histologic evidence of new collagen formulation using platelet rich plasma in skin rejuvenation: a prospective controlled clinical study. Ann Dermatol 2016;28: 718–24.

28. Redaelli A, Romano D, Marciano A. Face and neck revitalization with platelet-rich plasma (PRP): clinical outcome in a series of 23 consecutively treated patients. J Drugs Dermatol 2010;9:466–72.

29. Diaz-Ley B, Cuevast J, Alonso-Castro L, et al. Benefits of plasma rich in growth factors (PRGF) in skin photodamage: clinical response and histological assessment. Dermatol Ther 2015;28:258–63.

30. Sclafani AP, Saman M. Platelet-rich fibrin matrix for facial plastic surgery. Facial Plast Surg Clin North Am 2012;20:177–86, vi.

31. Ardakani MR, Moein HP, Beiraghdar M. Tangibility of platelet-rich fibrin matrix for nasolabial folds. Adv Biomed Res 2016;5:197.

32. Cameli N, Mariano M, Cordone I, et al. Autologous pure platelet-rich plasma dermal injections for facial skin rejuvenation: clinical, instrumental, and flow cytometry assessment. Dermatol Surg 2017;43: 826–35.

33. Hersant B, SidAhmed-Mezi M, Niddam J, et al. Efficacy of autologous platelet-rich plasma combined with hyaluronic acid on skin facial rejuvenation: a prospective study. J Am Acad Dermatol 2017;77: 584–6.

34. Kamakura T, Kataoka J, Maeda K, et al. Platelet-rich plasma with basic fibroblast growth factor for treatment of wrinkles and depressed areas of the skin. Plast Reconstr Surg 2015;136:931–9.

35. James IB, Coleman SR, Rubin JP. Fat, stem cells, and platelet-rich plasma. Clin Plast Surg 2016;43: 473–88.

36. Ersek RA, Chang P, Salisbury MA. Lipo layering of autologous fat: an improved technique with promising results. Plast Reconstr Surg 1998;101:820–6.

37. Liao HT, Marra KG, Rubin JP. Application of platelet-rich plasma and platelet-rich fibrin in fat grafting: basic science and literature review. Tissue Eng Part B Rev 2014;20:267–76.

38. Willemsen JC, van der Lei B, Vermeulen KM, et al. The effects of platelet-rich plasma on recovery time and aesthetic outcome in facial rejuvenation: preliminary retrospective observations. Aesthetic Plast Surg 2014;38:1057–63.

39. Rigotti G, Charles-de-Sa L, Gontijo-de-Amorim NF, et al. Expanded stem cells, stromal-vascular fraction, and platelet-rich plasma enriched fat: comparing results of different facial rejuvenation approaches in a clinical trial. Aesthetic Surg J 2016;36: 261–70.

40. Willemsen JCN, Van Dongen J, Spiekman M, et al. The addition of PRP to facial lipofilling: a double-blind placebo-controlled randomized trial. Plast Reconstr Surg 2018;141(2):331–43.

41. Gentile P, De Angelis B, Pasin M, et al. Adipose-derived stromal vascular fraction cells and platelet-rich plasma: basic and clinical evaluation for cell-based therapies in patients with scars on the face. J Craniofac Surg 2014;25:267–72.

42. Cervelli V, Gentile P, Scioli MG, et al. Application of platelet-rich plasma in plastic surgery: clinical and in vitro evaluation. Tissue Eng Part C Methods 2009;15:625–34.

43. Fontdevila J, Guisantes E, Martinez E, et al. Double-blind clinical trial to compare autologous fat grafts versus autologous fat grafts with PDGF: no effect of PDGF. Plast Reconstr Surg 2014;134:219e–30e.

44. Lee JW, Kim BJ, Kim MN, et al. The efficacy of autologous platelet rich plasma combined with ablative carbon dioxide fractional resurfacing for acne scars: a simultaneous split-face trial. Dermatol Surg 2011; 37:931–8.

45. Gawdat HI, Hegazy RA, Fawzy MM, et al. Autologous platelet rich plasma: topical versus intradermal after fractional ablative carbon dioxide laser treatment of atrophic acne scars. Dermatol Surg 2014; 40:152–61.

46. Hui Q, Chang P, Guo B, et al. The clinical efficacy of autologous platelet-rich plasma combined with ultra-pulsed fractional CO2 laser therapy for facial rejuvenation. Rejuvenation Res 2017;20:25–31.

47. Shin MK, Lee JH, Lee SJ, et al. Platelet-rich plasma combined with fractional laser therapy for skin rejuvenation. Dermatol Surg 2012;38:623–30.

Microneedling with Biologicals
Advantages and Limitations

Diane Irvine Duncan, MD

KEYWORDS

- Microneedling • Dermaceuticals • RF needling • Fractional laser

KEY POINTS

- Microneedling is a recently popular procedure for aesthetic skin enhancement.
- Uptake of drugs and biologic agents is enhanced when microchannels are created in the dermis.
- Thermal needling creates a subdermal sponge; therefore, topical agent uptake is magnified up to 10 times over nonthermal needling.
- The Food and Drug Administration position notes that topical agents intended to change the structure or function of the skin are drugs and should be regulated.

INTRODUCTION

The use of microneedling to introduce topical agents into the dermis is a rapidly growing and popular skin treatment. New devices and techniques offer nearly painless treatment sessions with little temporary deformity or down time. In most cases, these treatments are cost effective and take under 30 minutes to perform. Recent dermatology and aesthetic medicine–based meetings have focused on this hot topic, as controversy over the best way to treat the target area, the best topical agents to use in certain conditions, and concerns regarding Food and Drug Administration (FDA) regulation of this emerging minimally invasive treatment category arise. Other points of controversy include the relative efficacy of cold versus thermal microneedling, and efficacy of topical platelet-rich plasma (PRP) versus acellular extracted growth factors or stem cell–targeted small proteins. Difficulty in measuring efficacy of these treatments compounds the confusion regarding claims made in marketing and advertising various skin treatments. Variables in manufacturing and processing these topical

agents result in products that cannot be accurately compared. Histologic analysis does not always reflect clinical outcome. Patient satisfaction measurements, and measurements of skin tone and texture and not standardized enough to accurately quantify outcomes.

HISTORY

The use of topical biological agents dates back to ancient times, when honey[1] was commonly used for wound healing, as an antimicrobial, a binder for cosmetics, and a humectant and wrinkle retardant. In the 1950s, Michel Pistor[2] developed a method of mesotherapy in which needles were used to pierce the skin multiple times as a method of introducing drugs or various other substances. After mesotherapy needling, topical agents were applied for purposes ranging from hair regeneration to treatment of hypertension, gout, infertility, and endocrine disorders.[3,4] Although the proposed mechanism of action of plant based stem cells is not scientifically explained, many cosmetic companies[5–7] maintain that these topical agents

Disclosure Statement: Consultant for DefenAge, InMode.
Private Practice, 1701 East Prospect Road, Fort Collins, CO 80525, USA
E-mail address: dduncan@drdianeduncan.com

Facial Plast Surg Clin N Am 26 (2018) 447–454
https://doi.org/10.1016/j.fsc.2018.06.006

stimulate the development of new collagen or skin cells. The use of adipose-derived stem cells for aesthetic use has been curtailed by regulation by the FDA.[8] Another more recent introduction is the application of topical bone marrow–derived stem cells that can be obtained from multiple sources.[9,10] The development of targeted peptides or small proteins to stimulate inherently existing stem cells was reported in 2015.[11]

MATERIALS AND METHODS
Devices

There are several types of microneedling devices that create blunt or sharp injuries to the skin, usually into the epidermis. There are hand-held stamping devices, dermarollers, and motorized devices that either stamp or glide.[12,13] Needle length varies. A popular length is 0.5 mm because it seems well tolerated, especially with prior application of topical anesthetic. Probably the most common needle length used is 1.0 mm. Nonthermal, or cold, microneedling is commonly practiced in spa-level settings. Thermal needling usually implements device that use radiofrequency (RF) energy. Common devices are bipolar or multipolar. The Jeisys device (Intracel, Seoul, Korea) is bipolar and is designed primarily to treat Asian skin. Energy is applied between the needles, creating a strong ablative field.[14] The InMode device is bipolar, and the energy is applied through the needles across 2 poles.[15] The focus with this device is on tightening. Other RF needling devices include the Infini (Lutronic [Billerica, MA]) and the Intensif (Endymed [New York, NY]). RF needling devices are commonly used to treat acne scarring in patients with darker skin types.[16,17] Thermal microneedling devices generally cost more than cold, or nonthermal, devices. Several offer multiple depths of fractional injury, with varying degrees of temporary deformity and different lengths of healing time required. Although many thermal needling devices are FDA approved, currently no nonthermal microneedling devices have obtained FDA approval. Another thermal device that also creates needle-like epidermal and superficial dermal injury is the fractional laser.[18] Both CO_2 and erbium lasers have been used in creating microchannels for dermaceutical application.[19]

Methods

There are 3 basic techniques for nonthermal microneedling. The least expensive devices are dermarollers, which use small needles fixed on a rolling cylinder. These are popular for personal use. Concerns about transmission of blood-borne pathogens exist if these rollers were to be used on multiple patients. Stamping devices, such as Thermage (Solta Medical, Pleasanton, CA), Viora (Viora, New York, NY), and ProCell (Santa Ana, California), use blunt or sharp needles attached to a disposable tip that is attached to a separate device. The tips are discarded after each use and are mechanically designed so that cross-contamination is unlikely. Gliding devices, such as Dermapen (Terrey Hills, NSW, Australia), Rejuvapen (Jacksonville Beach, FLA), and Micro-Pen (Honeoye Falls, NY), contain a smaller tip with vibrating needles that are stroked across the surface of the skin. Down time typically is less with rolling or stamping devices than with gliding microneedling machines.

Techniques with RF-based thermal needles are more standardized. With some devices, tips with different needle lengths can be used to treat superficially and/or deep. The Jeisys device has the ability to vary needle depths in a single tip. Needles can be uncoated, so that energy is delivered along the entire needle, or they can be coated, so that energy is only released well below the epidermis. These devices use a stamping technique. Energy used can vary greatly. When treating with RF needling plus a topical, in most cases, lower energy settings are recommended. Some drugs and biologic agents can magnify the thermal injury created with the device. As yet, there are no safe transdermal dose recommendations for topical agents used in combination with microneedling. The number of passes or stacked pulses should also be conservative for the same reason.

Techniques with fractional laser are also fairly standard. Generally, 100 μm to 150 μm is a good starting point as far as depth, with 5% to 10% density because an extremely dense pattern may cause drug toxicity, delayed healing, or the appearance of a burn. One pass to a maximum of 2 passes are generally sufficient in a treatment region prior to topical application. This type of treatment would not be recommended for darker skin types.

A spilt face study was performed in order to see if alternative topical dermaceuticals could stack up to PRP. Given the premise that PRP improves skin quality,[20] a pilot study was performed to evaluate the difference in outcome between PRP as a biologic agent and a defensin-based serum in a split-face study performed in 2017. Ten patients were treated. Three patients had Halo (Sciton, Palo Alto, CA) hybrid fractional laser prior to topical agent application, 3 underwent Fractora (Inmode, Lake Forest, CA) radiofrequency-assisted needling, and 4 had nonthermal microneedling prior to application of each agent. The device used for cold microneedling was ProCell, which uses a stamping rather than a gliding technique. RF needling was performed with the Fractora device. The fractional laser used was the Halo hybrid erbium/sublative from Sciton. PRP resource was Regen Lab (Lausanne, Switzerland). Defensin serum was obtained from DefenAge (Carlsbad, California).

After both informed consent and study consent was obtained, each patient drew a straw to determine the facial location of PRP application and defensin serum application post-treatment. Topical local anesthetic (Betacaine Tetracaine Lidocaine [BLT] Cornell Pharmacy, Denver, Colorado) was applied for 30 minutes prior to treatment. In group 1, the ProCell device with a 0.5-mm tip was used to treat the face with 3 passes. In group 2, the Halo hybrid fractional laser was used to treat the face with 2 passes. In group 3, the Fractora device was used to treat the face with 2 passes. PRP, prepared prior to treatment, was applied topically to the designated side of the treated face immediately post-treatment. Defensin serum was applied 30 minutes post-treatment on the opposite side. The patient was instructed to leave both topicals on the face until the next morning, when the face could be washed with a gentle cleanser. Patients were instructed to resume their normal skin care regime.

Patients were seen in follow-up at 1 week and 6 weeks post-treatment. Standardized photographs were taken at 6 weeks. To better quantify the results, high-resolution standardized photographs (FotoFinder, Columbia, Maryland) were sent to MS Clinical research in Bangalore, India, where a computerized analysis was undertaken.

RESULTS

Surprisingly, simple microneedling can produce visible changes in the appearance of the skin's surface (**Fig. 1**). The ease and speed of application of topical biological agents plus patients' desire for the most improvement possible make this add-on procedure easy and cost-effective. The application of simple biological agents, such as hyaluronic acid (HA), after microneedling can create a marked change in both clinical and histologic appearance of the skin (**Fig. 2**). Adding a bone marrow–derived mesenchymal stem cell preparation (MicroGlide GF [Eclipse, The Colony, Texas]) plus HA seems to give even more benefit (**Fig. 3**). Use of a defensin-based serum (DefenAge) after microneedling can create remarkable improvement in skin quality with a single treatment (**Fig. 4**). In the split-face patients, all saw some improvement. Analysis of post-treatment photographs showed more improvement in fine lines, redness, and pigment with thermal microneedling than with nonthermal microneedling, although the sample size was too small to be statistically significant. One patient, treated with RF needling plus topical PRP and defensin serum, is shown in **Fig. 5**. A close look shows that the defensin serum treatment side showed a bit more clinical improvement than the PRP-treated side. Quantitative analysis confirms this impression, because the wrinkle measurement pixel value reduction is greater on the defensin side in this single case. This type of measurement has great value because the basic wrinkle measurements are not the same on both sides prior to treatment. In **Fig. 6**, a patient with severe rosacea has been treated with Halo fractional laser plus PRP on the right and defensing serum on the left. After treatment, both sides showed dramatic improvement, although the defensing treated side was quantitatively a bit better. With any combination treatment, it is difficult to definitively say which part of the treatment had the most influence on outcome. Thermal needling alone creates significant improvement.

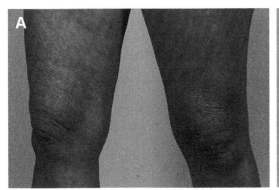 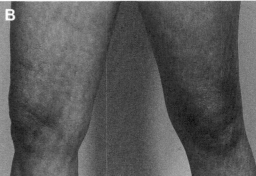

Fig. 1. (*A*) A 44-year-old patient before treatment. (*B*) One month after nonthermal microneedling treatment.

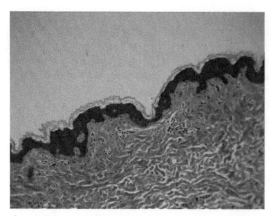

Fig. 2. Hematoxylin-eosin stain showing histology 2 weeks after microneedling plus topical HA application. Note a sustained effect on the stratum corneum. (hematoxylin-eosin, original magnification ×100).

DISCUSSION

Topical biological agents commonly used with microneedling include HA,[21] PRP,[22] cultured or extracted bone marrow–derived mesenchymal cells,[23] vitamin C,[24] Kojic acid, and small peptides that target existing banks of quiescent stem cells. Many other products are applied to treated skin; none is FDA approved for this purpose. The FDA states that if a topical product is used on injured skin for the purpose of changing the structure or function of the skin, it becomes a drug, therefore subject to FDA regulation.[25] The uptake of these drugs through damaged skin can be upward of 10 times the systemic concentration over those taken orally or applied to intact skin. Currently, no published studies address the potential toxicity of topical agents applied to skin treated with either

microneedling or thermal needling. Haak and colleagues[26] have done studies that show increased uptake of dermaceutical compounds after microneedling. Kalluri and colleagues[27] note that nonthermal microchannels close at about 4 hours to 5 hours postinjury. Oleson[28,29] note that although nonthermal needling channels close after several hours when a fibrin plug is formed, thermal needling creates an injury similar to a subepidermal sponge. The vehicle type of the topical agent directly affects the degree of uptake. Gel-like substances are somewhat inhibited due to their physical properties, whereas thinner liquids seem better absorbed. This study also noted that the character of the coagulation zone (CZ) surrounding the needling injury directly affects uptake. Although no CZ (0 μm) and a large CZ (80 μm) seemed to limit topical agent uptake, a CZ of 20 μm enhances uptake significantly in CO_2 fractional lasered skin. Settings used to achieve this optimal uptake were a treatment depth of 150 μm and a pattern density of 5%. The investigators noted that a thin CZ of 20 μm seemed most efficacious. The timing of topical application is important.[2] Fluorescence intensity of introduced topical agents was highest when the agent was applied within 30 minutes of treatment. This study used optical coherence tomography to show that 100% of the microchannels were open at 30 minutes, 75% were open at 6 hours, and only 3% were open at 24 hours to 48 hours.

FOOD AND DRUG ADMINISTRATION CONTROVERSY

In 2017 the FDA issued a bulletin entitled, "Regulatory Considerations for Microneedling Devices."[30] The document states that the recommendations are draft suggestions, not for implementation at this time. The classification of microneedling devices into 2 categories is set forth. Those devices intended to treat a disease state or to change the structure or function of the living skin layers (anything other than stratum corneum) are considered a device subject to FDA regulation. If the microneedling device is intended only to improve luminosity, exfoliate, or give the skin a smoother look and feel, it is not considered a device that needs FDA approval. Claims for treating acne, wrinkles, and alopecia infer an intent to change the structure and function of the skin. Also, any device that touts collagenesis, neovascularization, or improved wound healing is also subject to FDA approval through the (510)K process. The FDA document notes that a combination product

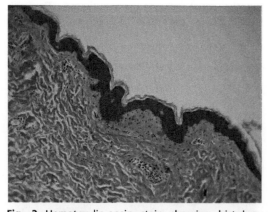

Fig. 3. Hematoxylin-eosin stain showing histology 2 weeks after microneedling plus HA and bone marrow–derived cultured stem cell application. (hematoxylin-eosin, original magnification ×100).

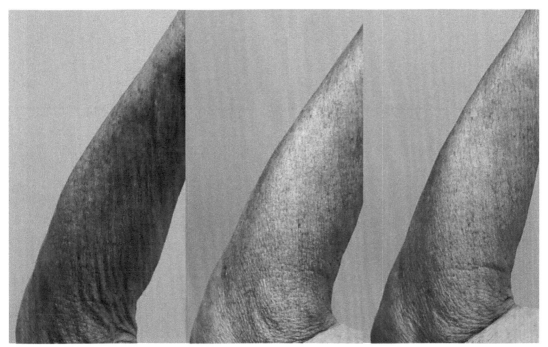

Fig. 4. (*Left*) A 62-year-old patient with solar elastosis and wrinkling, poor skin tone. (*Middle*) Thirty minutes after nonthermal microneedling and application of defensin serum. (*Right*) Appearance 1 month post-treatment.

might include topical agents applied before, during, or after microneedling, which could include "creams, ointments, gels, vitamin solutions, drugs, or blood products (eg, platelet-richplasma)." These products would be subject to regulation by the Center for Drug Evaluation and Research or the Center for Biologics Evaluation and Research. Combination products are any topical or injectable product supplied by the company with the microneedling device, sold by the microneedling device company, or any product for which instructions for use in combination with microneedling might be provided by the company. FDA representatives have publicly stated that dermaceuticals applied to cold or thermally needled skin represent drugs, because they are intended to change the structure or function of the skin.[25] To date, no action has been taken by the FDA to formally regulate these chemical or biological agents, but it is fairly likely that an opinion on this type of application will be rendered in the not so distant future.

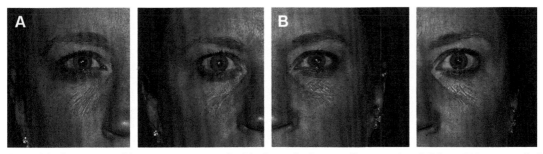

Fig. 5. (*A*) This 54-year-old patient was treated with thermal microneedling over her full face. PRP was applied immediately post-treatment to the right face. Computer-based fine line analysis shows an improvement of 389 units in the infraorbital region. (*B*). Same patient treated with thermal RF needling on the left side, followed by application of defensin serum 30 minutes post-treatment. Wrinkle reduction improvement index was 501 on this side.

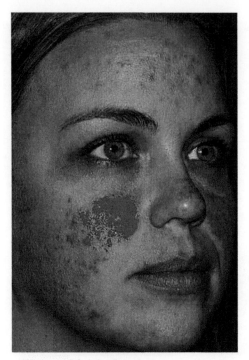
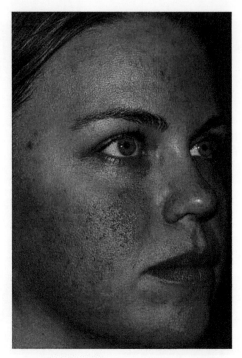

35 year old right face before treatment   Patient 6 weeks post Halo plus PRP

Redness

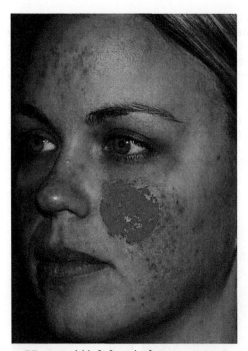
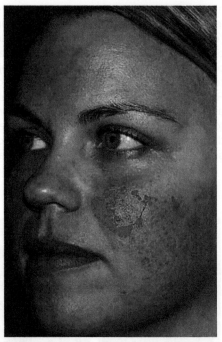

35 year old left face before treatment   Patient 6 weeks post Halo and defensin

Fig. 6. This 35-year-old patient had severe bullous rosacea. She was treated with Halo hybrid erbium and sublative laser over her full face. The right side was treated with PRP immediately post-treatment. The left side was treated with defensin-based serum 30 minutes post-treatment. The right side showed a quantitative redness reduction of 2207 units. The left side showed a 2945-unit improvement. The advantage of this quantitative method rests in its ability to measure a preexisting deformity, then measure improvement based on objective evaluation.

SUMMARY

Although application of topical agents on skin treated with thermal or nonthermal needling or fractional laser is common, controversy regarding safety and efficacy is strong. Measurements of safety and efficacy are mainly subjective, and reports of complications are not unusual. Because there is no current method of measuring drug uptake in the epidermis or dermis, the application of a safe dose is impossible to determine. In effect, the current trend of applying topical compounds on needled skin is similar to the mesotherapy era, in which a hodgepodge of agents never intended for dermal use was applied to needled skin without regard to toxicity or efficacy.

REFERENCES

1. Burlando B, Cornara L. Honey in dermatology and skin care: a review. J Cosmet Dermatol 2013 Dec; 12(4):306–13.
2. Pistor M. What is mesotherapy? Chir Dent Fr 1976; 46(288):59–60.
3. Rotunda A, Kolodney MS. Mesotherapy and phosphatidylcholine injections: historical clarification and review. Dermatol Surg 2006;32:465–80.
4. Le Coz J. History of mesotherapy. 2005. Available at: http://www.mesotherapyworldwide.com/images/pdf/AJM_Vol_3_200511_40.pdf. Accessed November 21, 2009.
5. Korkina GL, Mayer W, de Luca C. Meristem plant cells as a sustainable Source of Redox Actives for Skin Rejuvenation. Biomolecules 2017;7(2):40.
6. Trehan S, Michniak-Kohn B, Beri K. Plant stem cells in cosmetics: current trends and future directions [review]. Future Sci OA 2017;3(4):FSO226.
7. Beri K, Milgraum SS. Neocollagenesis in deep and superficial dermis by combining fractionated Q-Switched ND: YAG 1,064-nm with topical plant stem cell extract and N-acetyl glucosamine: open case series. J Drugs Dermatol 2015;14(11):1342–6.
8. Available at: https://www.fda.gov/downloads/biologicsbloodvaccines/guidancecomplianceregulatoryinformation/guidances/tissue/ucm062592.pdf. Accessed December 28, 2017.
9. Kwon TR, Oh CT, Choi EJ, et al. Conditioned medium from human bone marrow-derived mesenchymal stem cells promotes skin moisturization and effacement of wrinkles in UVB-irradiated SKH-1 hairless mice. Photodermatol Photoimmunol Photomed 2016;32(3):120–8.
10. Motegi SI, Ishikawa O. Mesenchymal stem cells: The roles and functions in cutaneous wound healing and tumor growth. J Dermatol Sci 2017;86(2):83–9.
11. Lough D, Dai H, Yang M, et al. Stimulation of the follicular bulge LGR5+ and LGR6+ stem cells with the gut-derived human alpha defensin 5 results in decreased bacterial presence, enhanced wound healing, and hair growth from tissues devoid of adnexal structures. Plast Reconstr Surg 2013; 132(5):1159–71.
12. Badran MM, Kuntsche J, Fahr A. Skin penetration enhancement by a microneedle device (Dermaroller®) in vitro: Dependency on needle size and applied formulation. Eur J Pharm Sci 2009;36:511–23.
13. Singh A, Yadav S. Microneedling: advances and widening horizons. Indian Dermatol Online J 2016; 7(4):244–54.
14. Available at: www.jeisys.com/2016/product/intracel/. Accessed December 17, 2017.
15. Loesch MM, Somani A, Kingsley MM, et al. Skin resurfacing procedures: new and emerging options. Clin Cosmet Investig Dermatol 2014;7: 231–41.
16. Cho SI, Chung BY, Choi MG, et al. Evaluation of the clinical efficacy of fractional radiofrequency microneedle treatment. In acne scars and large facial pores. Dermatol Surg 2012;38: 1017–24.
17. Connolly D, Vu HL, Mariwalla H, et al. Acne scarring—pathogenesis, evaluation, and treatment options. J Clin Aesthet Dermatol 2017;10(9): 12–23.
18. Wenande E, Erlendsson AM, Haedersdal M. Opportunities for laser-assisted drug delivery in the treatment of cutaneous disorders. Semin Cutan Med Surg 2017;36(4):192–201.
19. Ibrahim O, Wenande E, Hogan S, et al. Challenges to laser-assisted drug delivery: applying theory to clinical practice. Lasers Surg Med 2017. https://doi.org/10.1002/lsm.22769.
20. Hersant B, SidAhmed-Mezi M, Niddam J, et al. Efficacy of autologous platelet-rich plasma combined with hyaluronic acid on skin facial rejuvenation: a prospective study. J Am Acad Dermatol 2017; 77(3):584–6.
21. Iriarte C, Awosika O, Rengifo-Pardo M, et al. Review of applications of microneedling in dermatology. Clin Cosmet Investig Dermatol 2017;10: 289–98.
22. Abuaf OK, Yildiz H, Baloglu H, et al. Histologic evidence of new collagen formulation using platelet rich plasma in skin rejuvenation: a prospective controlled clinical study. Ann Dermatol 2016;28(6): 718–24.
23. Wang N, Liu H, Li X, et al. Activities of MSCs derived from transgenic mice seeded on ADM scaffolds in wound healing and assessment by advanced optical techniques. Cell Physiol Biochem 2017;42(2): 623–39.

24. Mehta-Ambalal SR. Neocollagenesis and neoelasti-nogenesis: from the laboratory to the clinic. J Cutan Aesthet Surg 2016;9(3):145–51.

25. Available at: https://www.fda.gov/drugs/information ondrugs/ucm079436.htm. Accessed December 28, 2017.

26. Haak CS, Hannibal J, Paasch U, et al. Laser-induced thermal coagulation enhances skin uptake of topically applied compounds. Lasers Surg Med 2017;49(6):582–91.

27. Kalluri H, Kolli CS, Banga AK. Characterization of microchannels created by metal microneedles: formation and closure. AAPS J 2011;13(3): 473–81.

28. Olesen UH, Mogensen M, Haedersdal M. Vehicle type affects filling of fractional laser-ablated channels imaged by optical coherence tomography. Lasers Med Sci 2017;32(3): 679–84.

29. Banzhaf CA, Thaysen-Petersen D, Bay C, et al. Fractional laser-assisted drug uptake: Impact of time-related topical application to achieve enhanced delivery. Lasers Surg Med 2017;49(4): 348–54.

30. Available at: https://www.fda.gov/downloads/medical devices/deviceregulationandguidance/guidance documents/ucm575923.pdf. Accessed December 28, 2017.

Lasers, Microneedling, and Platelet-Rich Plasma for Skin Rejuvenation and Repair

Karam W. Badran, MD*, Vishad Nabili, MD

KEYWORDS

- Platelet-rich plasma • Microneedling • Facial rejuvenation • Laser therapy • Facial scar

KEY POINTS

- Skin resurfacing for rejuvenation and repair continues to evolve with the development of noninvasive or minimally invasive, surgical substitutes and adjuvants within facial plastic surgery.
- Restoring tone and reversing the effects of environmental and genetic aging through nonsurgical modalities have attracted a great deal of attention for their reduced downtime, risk of complication, and sufficient treatment outcomes.
- Advances in optical and laser therapy, microneedling, and platelet-rich plasma have reinvigorated research in wound repair and regenerative science.

INTRODUCTION

Skin resurfacing for the purpose of rejuvenation and repair continues to evolve with the development of noninvasive or minimally invasive surgical substitutes and adjuvants within facial plastic surgery. Restoring tone and reversing the effects of environmental and genetic aging through nonsurgical modalities have attracted a great deal of attention for their reduced downtime, risk of complication, and sufficient treatment outcomes. Advances in optical and laser therapy, microneedling, and platelet-rich plasma (PRP) have reinvigorated research in wound repair and regenerative science. This article summarizes each of these modalities alone and reviews the potential additive benefits of combining these treatments to optimize facial rejuvenation.

LASER THERAPY IN FACIAL REJUVENATION

Laser resurfacing has long been an effective treatment in improving skin tone and texture, re-establishing a more youthful skin appearance. Founded on the basis of selective photothermolysis, ablative carbon dioxide (CO_2) laser treatment allows for destruction of specific layers of the epidermis and dermis with a controlled depth of thermal injury (chromophore, 10,600 nm).[1] Thermal vaporization within the dermis induces remodeling with new collagen synthesis, contraction, and subsequent tone, with good to excellent reported results in the treatment of photoaging and scar.[2–6]

Although effective in skin repair, prolonged adverse events using pure CO_2 laser therapy are common, occurring in 10% to 15% of patients and lasting up to 4.5 months.[7] These posttreatment adverse events include: edema, erythema, crusting, herpes simplex virus infection, and dermatitis.[8] Additionally, patients may experience long lasting pigmentary changes and scarring. Less ablative, more superficial lasers (Er:YAG; 2940 nm) have been used, although they are less effective because of reduced dermal collagen

Disclosure Statement: None.
Division of Facial Plastic and Reconstructive Surgery, Department of Head and Neck Surgery, David Geffen School of Medicine, University of California, Los Angeles, 10833 Le Conte Avenue, CHS 62-237, Los Angeles, CA 90095, USA
* Corresponding author.
E-mail address: kbadran@mednet.ucla.edu

Facial Plast Surg Clin N Am 26 (2018) 455–468
https://doi.org/10.1016/j.fsc.2018.06.007
1064-7406/18/© 2018 Elsevier Inc. All rights reserved.

remodeling.[9] Ongoing efforts in balancing adverse symptoms with treatment efficacy have resulted in the development of a concept termed fractional photothermolysis (FP).

Fractional Photothermolysis

Fractional ablative technologies create microscopic thermal wounds, conservatively sparing tissue surrounding each wound.[10] Because of small regions of tissue injury surrounded by normal skin, a macroscopic treatment effect is tailored by the arrangement and shape of the microscopic treatment zones (MTZ). Additionally, recent interest in FP technology has resulted in investigations for its possible use as a topical drug delivery system.[11]

The dermal stimulation achieved by using ablative FP has allowed for the successful treatment of scars, rhytides, and photodamaged skin.[12,13] The greatest advantage of avoiding confluent epidermal damage, in contrast to pure ablative laser resurfacing, is the reported lower incidence of scarring and pigment changes, with reported hyperpigmentation rates of 30% in pure laser therapy.[12,14,15] Despite the reduction in adverse symptoms, post-treatment events still arise and include: acneiform eruptions, temporary hyperpigmentation, and persistent erythema, with an incidence of 13% to 17% in recent studies with long-term follow-up.[16–18] Investigations to further improve outcomes following fractional laser therapy have used PRP as a pretreatment and post-treatment adjuvant and are summarized in **Table 1**.

MICRONEEDLING IN FACIAL REJUVENATION

Unlike energy-based laser therapy, microneedling, also known as percutaneous collagen induction, relies on focused areas of mechanical injury to disrupt the dermal skin layer. The ensuing inflammatory and wound healing cascade is then triggered with the release of growth factors and subsequent collagen deposition.[28,29] Patient-derived histologic results have corroborated translational research with the up-regulation of transforming growth factor (TGF)-β1-3 and increased collagen and elastin deposition at 1-year follow up.[30–32] These encouraging results are clinically demonstrated in the treatment of acne scar, photodamage, skin rejuvenation, and androgenetic alopecia.[33–35] The use of combination topical products with needling seems to be a natural progression of this treatment modality. Given the endogenous growth factors found within platelet granules, we have reviewed the literature for possible improvements in outcome and reductions in adverse treatment symptoms (**Table 2**).

PLATELET-RICH PLASMA IN FACIAL REJUVENATION

PRP has recently garnered growing interest as an effective modality for acute and chronic wound repair in several surgical and medical fields.[41–44] Harboring growth factors and cytokines, PRP has been viewed as an elixir of youth. The ease with which it is harvested, grafted, and activated has resulted in wide ranging publications as an adjuvant to conventional treatment modalities. Through topical application or injection, PRP is aimed to replenish the depleted local levels of growth factors and propagate healing through a myriad of chemotactic pathways.[45–47] With similar parallels between wound healing and regeneration of aging skin, the potential to enhance recovery and improve results following skin resurfacing is promising.

Platelet-Rich Plasma: Role in Cutaneous Regeneration

Over the past two decades, a boon in literature attempting to maximize the intrinsic potential of platelet-derived growth factors has resulted in a better understanding of the biologic and molecular pathways for skin repair. Following activation, platelets release alpha-granules containing growth factors and cytokines including platelet-derived growth factor, TGFs, vascular endothelial growth factor, insulin-like growth factor, epidermal growth factor, and interleukin-1.[48,49] These signaling proteins are integral to the remodeling that occurs within the extracellular matrix during aging and repair. Several of the investigations used within this article, and original investigations using PRP alone, confirm the potential of PRP to induce and promote collagen synthesis, regulated by fibroblasts.[50,51] These include the ability to reverse the effects of collagenases, increase collagen levels, and decrease tissue inflammation.[52]

Skin Repair and Scar

Wound healing is initiated by the recruitment of circulating inflammatory cells to the wound site, initiating re-epithelialization, tissue contraction, and an angiogenic response. These processes are coordinated by locally released and locally acting growth factors that control cell growth and proliferation, namely: platelet-derived growth factor, vascular endothelial growth factor, TGF-β, and tissue inhibitor of metalloproteinases.[47] The remodeling that occurs following wound repair stimulates new collagen, elastin, and glycosaminoglycans.[53] These matrix components are diminished in aging skin and abnormally organized in scar formation.[54,55]

Table 1
Platelet-rich plasma adjuvant to laser therapy

Author, Year	Number of Patients Enrolled (M/F)	Condition Treated	Adjuvant Effect of PRP Investigated	Site Treated	Type of Resurfacing	PRP Delivery	Activated In Vitro (Y/N)	Timing of PRP	Treatment Interval and Duration	Control Group	Follow-up After Final Treatment	Objective Outcomes	Subjective Outcomes	Patient Survey	Histology
Na et al,[19] 2011	25	NA	Postlaser symptoms	Inner arm	FCL	Topical	Yes CaCl$_2$	Immediately following laser treatment	Laser: once	Saline topical	4 wk	SS reductions in waterloss, E-index, and M-index with PRP therapy compared with control group	Reduced erythema and pigmentation in PRP group	ND	H&E: thicker epidermis, more organized stratum corneum, higher density of collagen in PRP group
Lee et al,[20] 2011	10/4	Atrophic acne scar	Scar repair	Face	FCL	Intradermal	ND	Immediately following laser treatment	Laser: 1 tx/1 mo Duration: 2 tx	Split-face Saline injection	4 mo	SS reduction in E-index on Day 4	SS reduction in duration of tx symptoms: erythema, edema SS greater improvement in repair of scar	ND	ND
Shin et al,[21] 2012	0/22	Aging skin	Rejuvenation	Face	Fractional erbium laser	Topical	Yes CaCl$_2$	Immediately following laser treatment	Laser: 1 tx/4 wk Duration: 3 tx	Laser alone	1 mo	Roughness: SS decrease compared with baseline, not with control Elasticity: SS increase in control compared with PRP group Hydration: no SSD between groups E-index: SS reduction in PRP group compared with control M-index: no SSD between groups	Improved overall appearance in PRP group compared with control but no SSD	Improvements with PRP compared with control: skin texture (100% vs 58%), elasticity (92% vs 67%) No SSD compared with control in pain, or erythema scales	SS improvement compared with control in the number of fibroblasts, dermal-epidermal junction length, and average area fraction of collagen

(continued on next page)

Table 1
(continued)

Author, Year	Number of Patients Enrolled (M/F)	Condition Treated	Adjuvant Effect of PRP Investigated	Site Treated	Type of Resurfacing	PRP Delivery	Activated In Vitro (Y/N)	Timing of PRP	Treatment Interval and Duration	Control Group	Follow-up After Final Treatment	Objective Outcomes	Subjective Outcomes	Patient Survey	Histology
Gawdat et al,[22] 2013	12/18	Atrophic acne scar	Scar repair	Face	FCL	Intradermal and topical	Yes CaCl$_2$	Immediately following laser treatment	Laser: 1 tx/1 mo Duration: 3 tx	Split-face Saline injection	3 mo	Optical coherence tomography: SS greater improvement in scar depth with PRP than control	SS improvement with PRP compared with control in skin smoothness	SS reduction in side effects and downtime with PRP. PRP improved scar in >60% of patients, compared with 26.7% of control patients	ND
Kim and Gallo,[23] 2015	15	NA	Postlaser symptoms	Forearm	FCL	Subcutaneous	ND	Immediately following laser treatment	Laser: 1 tx	Saline injection	18 d	ND	SS reduction in erythema and edema compared with control	PRP improved posttreatment erythema (71%), edema (67%), pain (67%), and pruritus (89%)	ND
Faghihi et al,[24] 2016	4/12	Atrophic acne scar	Scar repair	Face	FCL	Intradermal	Yes CaCl$_2$	Immediately following laser treatment	Laser: 1 tx/1 mo Duration: 2 tx	Split-face Saline injection	4 mo	ND	PRP improved outcomes at 1 mo (68.8% vs 50%) and 5 mo (87.5% vs 68.8%) compared with control	PRP treatment improved outcomes at 1 mo (50% vs 31.2%) and 5 mo (56.2% vs 43.8%) compared with control	ND
Abdel Aal et al,[25] 2017	18/12	Atrophic acne scar	Scar repair	Face	FCL	Intradermal	Yes CaCl$_2$	Immediately following laser treatment	Laser: 1 tx/3–4 wk Duration: 2 tx	Split-face Laser alone	6 mo	ND	Blinded clinician scoring: SS improvement of scar, duration of laser symptoms, incidence of PIH, in PRP group compared with control	SS greater patient satisfaction with the PRP compared with control side	ND

Hui et al,[26] 2017	0/13	Aging skin	Rejuvenation	Face	FCL	Intradermal and topical	Yes CaGluc	Prelaser injection Postlaser topical	Laser: 1 tx/3 mo Duration: 3 tx	Split-face Saline injection and topical	3 mo	VISIA Complexion Analysis System: SS improvement in wrinkles, textures, and elasticity	Improvements in experimental group but not SSD compared with control	SS improvement in facial wrinkles, skin texture, and skin elasticity	ND
Min et al,[27] 2017	25	Atrophic acne scar	Scar repair	Face	FCL	Intradermal	Yes CaCl$_2$	Immediately following laser treatment	Laser: 1 tx/4 wk Duration: 2 tx	Split-face Saline injection	3 mo	SS reduction in E-index with PRP	SS improvement in IGA and ECCA scaring scores with combination therapy compared with control for all scar subtypes	SS higher patient satisfaction scores for PRP combination therapy at 7 and 84 d following treatment	SS increase in fibrogenetic molecules (c-myc, TIMP, HGF, p-AKT, collagen 1 and 3) with PRP; time and dose dependent

Manuscripts reviewed are listed. Study designs and results are summarized.

Abbreviations: CaGluc, calcium gluconate; ECCA, Echelle d'Evaluation clinique des Cicatrices d'acné; E-index, erythema index; FCL, fractional CO$_2$ laser; H&E, hematoxylin and eosin; IGA, Invesetigator's Global Assessment Scale; M-index, melanin index; NA, not applicable; ND, not disclosed; PIH, postinflammatory hyperpigmentation; SS, statistically significant; SSD, statistically significant difference; tx, treatment.

Table 2
Platelet-rich plasma adjuvant to microneedling therapy

Author, Year	Number of Patients Enrolled (M/F)	Condition Treated	Adjuvant Effect of PRP Investigated	Site Treated	Type of Resurfacing	PRP Delivery	Activated In Vitro (Y/N)	Timing of PRP	Treatment Interval and Duration	Control Group	Follow-up After Final Treatment	Objective Outcomes	Subjective Outcomes	Patient Survey	Histology
Chawla,[36] 2014	19/8	Atrophic acne scar	Scar repair	Face	MN	ND	Yes CaGluc	ND	MN: 1 tx/4 wk Duration: 4 tx	Split-face Topical vitamin C	4 wk	ND	Improved reduction in scar with PRP compared with vitamin C following microneedling	SS greater patient satisfaction in outcome with use of PRP than vitamin C	ND
Asif et al,[37] 2016	25/25	Atrophic acne scar	Scar repair	Face	MN	Intradermal PRP Topical fibrin gel	Yes CaCl$_2$	Following MN	MN: 1 tx/4 wk Duration: 3tx	Split-face Saline injection	3 mo	ND	SS improvement compared with baseline in both groups; greater frequency of excellent improvement with PRP than control	Greater patient satisfaction and frequency of excellent improvement with PRP than with control	ND
El-Domyati et al,[38] 2017	6/24	Atrophic acne scar	Scar repair	Face	MN	Topical	Yes CaGluc	Following MN	MN: 1 tx/2 wk Duration: 6 tx	Split-face MN alone	3 mo	ND	SS improvement of scar with PRP compared with control	ND	SS increase in epidermal thickness (54.91 ± 1.08 μm vs 50.93 ± 4.692 μm; $P = .032$); subjective increase in collagen density and organization

Ibrahim et al,[39] 2017	35	Atrophic acne scar	Scar repair	Face	MN	Topical	Yes	CaGluc	Following MN	MN: 1 tx/3 wk Duration: 4 tx	Split-face MN alone	3 mo and 12 mo	ND	SS reduction in symptom duration compared with control SS improvement compared with baseline, not to control	SS improvement compared with baseline but no SSD compared with control	ND
Ibrahim et al,[40] 2017	44/46	Atrophic scars	Scar repair	Any site	MN	Intradermal	Yes	$CaCl_2$	Alternating treatments biweekly	MN: 1 tx/2 wk PRP: 1 tx/2 wk Duration: $\leq$6 tx	MN alone PRP alone	3 mo	ND	SS improvement in scar repair compared with isolated treatments	SS greater patient satisfaction compared with either treatment alone	ND

Manuscripts reviewed are listed. Study designs and results are summarized.

Abbreviations: CaGluc, calcium gluconate; MN, microneedling; ND, not disclosed; SS, statistically significant; SSD, statistically significant difference; tx, treatment.

Aging Skin

Skin aging is a dynamic process attributed to intrinsic (genetically determined, age-associated factors) and extrinsic (environmental factors, ultraviolet radiation, cigarette smoke) processes.[56] A progressive, age-degeneration of connective tissue therefore may be hastened by overlapping molecular mechanisms.[57] Through the breakdown of collagen and elastin fibers, characteristic findings of photoaged and chronoaged skin are apparent and include loss of elasticity, atrophy, xerosis, and rhytides.[52,58] Histologically, these changes are demonstrated by reduced dermal thickness, number of papillae, collagen concentration, and vascularity.[59,60] These changes have been associated with reduced levels of growth factors and effective fibroblast function.[61]

Harvesting Techniques

A review of the methods and techniques of PRP harvest is found throughout this special edition of *Facial Plastics Clinics of North America*. In brief, the production of platelet concentrates for platelet-rich solutions begins with the harvest of peripheral venous blood. The collected specimen are centrifuged in one or two steps depending on the processing system.[62–64] The initial, low force, centrifugation allows the blood components to separate into three weight-dependent layers: (1) a top, supernatant, layer of platelet-poor plasma; (2) a "buffy coat" middle layer rich in platelets and containing white blood cells; and (3) a bottom, red blood cell layer.[65] The second step varies among the numerous protocols; however, in concept it is an attempt to discard the red blood cell and platelet-poor plasma layers. This is mediated by harvesting the platelet-poor plasma and buffy coat layers following the first centrifugation into a separate test tube. Under high centrifugal force, the platelet-rich layer and plasma supernatant are further separated improving the precipitant yield of platelets from plasma. The final liquid platelet suspension coined PRP aims to be enriched four to seven times that of whole blood to be considered therapeutically effective, shown to be approximately 1 to 1.5 million platelets/μL to induce mesenchymal stem cell proliferation.[66,67] Values greater than 1.5 million platelets/μL have been found to decrease angiogenesis.[68]

PLATELET-RICH PLASMA: AN ADJUVANT TO LASER THERAPY

Techniques aimed at reducing post-treatment adverse symptoms and improving outcomes following proven laser therapies have resulted in a natural progression of the use of PRP as an adjuvant to fractional laser therapy. Several recent studies have designed prospective short- and long-term investigations described in **Table 1**. This review summarizes their treatment outcomes.

Platelet-Rich Plasma Improves Postlaser Symptoms

Attempts at mitigating the adverse effects following fractional laser skin treatment have resulted in a myriad of patient-reported and clinician-validated studies. In the peritreatment acute setting, Lee and colleagues[20] found reductions in post-treatment laser symptoms when PRP was injected immediately following laser therapy. Four-days following fractional CO_2 laser (FCL) therapy, statistically significant differences in clinician-rated erythema scores were evident ($P<.01$) and the total duration of symptoms in the combination therapy group were significantly reduced; specifically, erythema (8.6 ± 2.0 days; $P = .047$), edema (6.1 ± 1.1 days; $P = .04$), and crusting (5.9 ± 1.1 days; $P = .04$).

Similar improvements in laser symptoms were achieved when PRP was applied before and following FCL. Where the total duration of erythema (8.31 ± 0.85 vs 9.08 ± 0.64 days; $P = .025$), edema (7.31 ± 0.48 vs 7.92 ± 0.64 days; $P = .013$), and crusting (7.15 ± 0.38 vs 7.85 ± 0.80 days; $P = .032$) were all reduced.[26] Reducing the duration and severity of laser therapy symptoms allows patients to return to their daily routine and reduce their post-procedure downtime as demonstrated by Gawdat and colleagues[22] with the use of PRP following photothermolysis (4.37 ± 1.52 days vs 2.27 ± 0.69 days; $P = .02$).

Although patient-reported outcomes and experience is one of the strongest indicators of treatment success, attempts to correlate objective data with patient experience have also been demonstrated. Following FCL treatment to the inner arm of 25 patients, Na and colleagues[19] noted significant reductions in transepidermal water loss, erythema index, and melanin index when evaluated by spectrophotometer and compared with the placebo-controlled group ($P<.05$). Similar reductions in erythema index and melanin index following topical facial application of PRP have been reported with the use of 1550-nm fractional erbium laser (erythema-index: 8.4 ± 0.9 vs 7.1 ± 0.9; $P = .005$; melanin-index: 32.9 ± 1.5 vs 31.1 ± 1.4; $P>.05$).[21]

The effects of PRP on postlaser hyperpigmentation are difficult to assess given the unpredictable nature of such adverse events. However, Abdel Aal and colleagues[25] reported five occurrences of postinflammatory hyperpigmentation in their study of patients with Fitzpatrick phototype 3 to 4. All five patients were observed in the control (non-PRP) group. Gawdat and colleagues[69] also demonstrated two events of postinflammatory hyperpigmentation in control, but not in the PRP-treated group.

Platelet-Rich Plasma Enhances Laser Rejuvenation Outcomes

Ablative fractional laser therapy is a current standard in the treatment of facial rhytides and photodamaged skin. The clinical outcomes are founded in the rapid healing and re-epithelialization that occurs between MTZ areas of tissue injury. Improving wound healing following skin damage may therefore result in improved treatment outcomes. This hypothesis has been tested in recent studies. Shin and colleagues[21] studied the effect of topical PRP applied to the facial cheek skin of 22 Korean women (Fitzpatrick scale 4 and 5) followed by fractional erbium laser. Patient-reported improvements in skin texture and elasticity were much higher than the saline-control group. A total of 100% of patients reported improvements in skin texture and 92% reported improvements in elasticity, compared with 58% and 67% in the control group, respectively. Biomechanical outcomes also demonstrated significant improvements of elasticity in the PRP group compared with control (10.3% vs 6.4%); however, they did not identify statistically significant differences in roughness, or hydration. The effect of injected intradermal PRP following FP was then investigated by Hui and colleagues.[26]

In their 2017 split-face, double-blinded, saline-placebo controlled study, Hui and colleagues[26] injected PRP and saline into opposing sides of the periorbital and forehead skin of 17 Fitzpatrick 3 and 4 women. Following FCL treatment, topical PRP and saline was applied to the experimental and control sides, respectively. Over a 3-month three-treatment duration, VISIA Complexion Analysis System (Canfield Imaging Systems, Fairfield, NJ) recorded objective age-related skin changes on each side of the patient's face. Following clinician ranking, the experimental side found significant improvements in skin wrinkles (1.72 ± 0.58 and 1.94 ± 0.55; $P = .145$), texture (0.99 ± 0.33 and 1.21 ± 0.42; $P = .010$), and elasticity (1.41 ± 0.43 and 1.54 ± 0.47; $P = .026$) compared with the contralateral face. Patients, blinded to the experimental side of their face, found significant improvements with PRP injection in facial wrinkles ($P = .039$), skin texture ($P = .039$), and skin elasticity ($P = .040$).

Platelet-Rich Plasma Enhances Laser Atrophic Scar Treatment

Fractional laser therapy has significantly remodeled the depressed and disorganized floor of atrophic scars through elevation of the collagenous dermal matrix.[70,71] Given the natural growth factors found in PRP, combination therapy may aid in improving laser scar treatment. Gawdat and colleagues[22] prospectively investigated the combined efficacy and safety of FCL with PRP in a randomized split-face comparative single-blind clinical trial in the treatment of atrophic acne scars with that of FCL alone. At 6-month follow-up, faces treated with PRP (intradermal or topical) following laser therapy demonstrated significantly greater improvements in scar depth measured by optical coherence tomography (28.9 ± 8.3 μm vs 48.8 ± 16.4 μm; $P = .01$), increased patient satisfaction (60% vs 27%), and reductions in postlaser adverse symptoms and down-time ($P = .02$) compared with the saline-controlled group. Clinician-graded outcomes have also demonstrated subjectively improved outcomes for the use of atrophic acne scar at 4 months.[20]

Platelet-Rich Plasma Imparts Favorable Molecular, Cellular, and Tissue Remodeling

Ablative fractional laser therapy resurfaces skin through tissue contraction in areas of MTZ. Several studies have demonstrated improvements in dermal thickness, neocollagenesis, and collagen contraction following laser therapy. The use of PRP may supplement these favorable histologic outcomes. Following 1550-nm fractional erbium laser treatment, Shin and colleagues[21] applied topical PRP and analyzed biopsy specimens 1 month following treatment. Cheek skin sites demonstrated significantly greater changes in the number of fibroblasts formed (delta +65.4% vs delta −19.4%), dermal-epidermal junction length (delta +67% vs delta +46.9%), and fraction of collagen formed (delta +2.8% vs delta −24.3%) compared with laser alone. Na and colleagues[19] found similarly positive histologic results 4 weeks following combination therapy when pretreated with PRP. Their study demonstrated a thicker epidermis layer, more organized stratum corneum layer, and higher collagen density.

Further investigation of skin with immunohistochemistry has demonstrated significantly increased molecular concentrations of fibrinogenic molecules with the use of PRP following laser therapy.[27] A positive time-dependent (4 week) response of protein cytokines and collagen was noted, specifically of TGF-β, epidermal growth factor receptor, tissue inhibitor of metalloproteinases, and collagen 1 and

3. Additionally, in vitro studies of irradiated fibroblast cells demonstrated more rapid recovery and increased proliferation at 24 hours when cultured in PRP compared with serum alone.[27]

PLATELET-RICH PLASMA AS AN ADJUVANT TO MICRONEEDLING

Considered a noninvasive device, microneedling has a low rate of post-treatment adverse symptoms. When present, these include: erythema, pinpoint bleeding, transient crusting, and localized edema, all of which typically resolve within 72 hours.[33,72] Histologic examination taken 24 hours after therapy demonstrates an intact epidermis and no change in melanocyte number, resulting in limited downtime and minimal risk of dyspigmentation.[28] The most severe post-treatment complication has been associated with the use of topical cosmeceuticals, specifically vitamin C and post-treatment granuloma formation.[73] Given the autogenous harvest of PRP the likelihood of such hypersensitive reactions is further diminished.

Platelet-Rich Plasma Improves Postmicroneedling Symptoms

Ibrahim and colleagues[39] prospectively studied the effects of topical PRP following microneedling in a split-face study of 35 individuals with mild to moderate acne scores 2 to 4 (Goodman-Baron scoring).[74,75] Their study demonstrated significantly reduced durations of erythema and edema on the side treated with skin needling followed by topical PRP (4.3 vs 6.2 days and 1.05 vs 3.3 days; $P<.001$). Similar subjective results were found by El-Domyati and colleagues[38] with early resolution in erythema, edema, and crusting in combination therapy. However, in a 90-patient prospective study, Ibrahim and colleagues[40] demonstrated greater severity of erythema in patients receiving intradermal PRP following microneedling than control groups, which consisted of PRP alone and needling alone ($P<.001$); however, duration and timing of symptom evaluation were not documented.

Platelet-Rich Plasma Improves Microneedling Outcomes in Atrophic Scar

Microneedling has most extensively been studied for acne scar treatment, with a recent systematic review demonstrating moderate efficacy among 10 heterogeneously designed investigations.[33] The ability to remodel atrophic scars is founded in the ability to induce neocollagenesis within the papillary dermis and epithelium.[72] However, scar type seems to be a factor because deep-seated atrophic ice pick scars are found to be less responsive than boxcar or rolling scars with microneedling.[33,40,76] Given the ease with which topical therapies may be transcutaneously delivered, and the low risk of hypersensitivity in autologous PRP, several studies have investigated the augmented effect of needling with platelet-rich concentrates.

In the earliest investigation, Chawla[36] designed a split-face prospective 4-week trial of microneedling and PRP in 27 patients with mild to severe atrophic acne scar. The study found PRP treatment to increase the number of "excellent" responders (18.5% vs 7%), whereas those treated with vitamin C incurred a greater frequency of "poor" improvement results (37% vs 22.2%). El-Domyati and colleagues[38] followed microneedling with topical PRP in a 30-patient split-face trial for atrophic acne scars. When compared with Derma Roller (Skin Tech Pharma Group, Pla de l'Estany, Spain) alone, the PRP group demonstrated significantly improved clinician-rated outcomes at 3-month follow-up (64.87 ± 28.67 vs 29.12 ± 22.52; $P = .015$) compared with control outcomes; no difference was found between the PRP and the trichloroacetic acid experimental group. When comparing all forms of atrophic scars (acne and traumatic) Ibrahim and colleagues[40] found a significantly greater improvement with PRP and Dermapen treatment compared with PRP or Dermapen (Terrey Hills, NSW, Australia) alone (chi-square test, 20.58; $P<.001$). On subgroup analysis, boxcar and ice pick acne scars demonstrated greater response than rolling acne scars ($P<.028$); however, nonacne scars had a greater response to treatment than acne scars ($P<.023$). Furthermore, a significant negative correlation between age of patient and duration of scar with response to treatment was also identified, indicating that younger patients with new scars showed higher response to treatment than patient with old scars. Patient satisfaction has also been reviewed noting consistently greater improvements with PRP therapy than without.[36,37,40]

Platelet-Rich Plasma Influences Postmicroneedling Histology

Microneedling alone has demonstrated increased epidermal thickness and stimulation of neocollagenesis with improvements in collagen organization and bundle patterns.[30–32] The investigations detailed in this article have all demonstrated improvements in skin thickness and collagen bundling when histology is available for combination and control groups. El-Domyati and co-workers[38] assessed histologic features 3 months following 6 treatments with microneedling and PRP (applied topically immediately following microneedling). All specimens demonstrated improvements compared with baseline; however, combination PRP therapy significantly increased epidermal thickness greater than needling alone (54.91 ± 1.08 μm vs 50.93 ± 4.692 μm; $P = .032$). Combination therapy also demonstrated an increase in deposition of more organized and parallel collagen bundles compared with control. The thicker epidermal layer has also demonstrated a greater numbers of rete ridges, and a greater concentration of elastic fibers, compared with baseline and needling alone.[40]

DISCUSSION

The potential of using an autogenous source of easily attainable growth factors to stimulate cellular regeneration, restore youth, and remodel scar has contributed to a growing number of clinical investigations. As an adjunct to laser and needling therapies, the topical and intradermal application of PRP to skin traumatized by mechanical and thermal microchannels seems to be feasible with no added side effects. Overall, PRP may be an effective means of enhancing wound healing, reducing transient unwanted effects, improving skin tightening, and delivering greater patient satisfaction to traditional modalities alone. All histologic studies reviewed demonstrate a greater concentration of organized collagen bundles with a thicker epidermal layer when compared with control groups. However, there exists only a small number of controlled clinical trials that provide evidence of its use in combination with long-standing methods of rejuvenation. Furthermore, wound healing is a dynamic process that occurs over long periods of time. Caution should be exercised when evaluating the results of each of these studies because the study design, treatment schedule, and patient population are heterogenous.

Research of novel modalities to improve outcomes over established technologies requires the standardization of current research endeavors. In facial plastic surgery, this may be difficult because there is no single set of treatment parameters that can be used in most patients to achieve a predicted outcome; skin varies among anatomic locations and patient background. Regarding PRP, known variations exist in platelet yield, kit manufacturer, and efficiencies between centrifuge system.[77–81] Documentation of these known confounders was found to be a critical limitation of current PRP research by Frautschi and colleagues,[41] noting inaccurate description of PRP composition, dosing, activation, and the use of subjective outcome measures. Additionally, the broad variation in cause, duration, and severity of scar and aged skin, Fitzpatrick phototype, duration of treatment used, and scheduling of treatment interval between each study cohort limits the ability to summarize the overall positive results from each of these studies independently.

Standardization of treatment-dosing protocols, site/area of injection, and injection technique are areas of future investigation. Additional randomized clinical trials with reproducible methods and those contrasting the effects of post-treatment cosmeceuticals will aid in powering larger cohort analyses with reduced study heterogeneity. Further evidence for the establishment of PRP as a supplement to traditional methods of skin rejuvenation and repair is needed to elucidate the therapeutic mechanism and optimal dosing by which PRP rejuvenates skin. Despite additional needed research, PRP has shown significant potential as a stand-alone or combined therapy along with laser or microneedling techniques to optimize facial rejuvenation.

REFERENCES

1. Anderson RR, Parrish JA. Selective photothermolysis: precise microsurgery by selective absorption of pulsed radiation. Science 1983;220(4596):524–7. Available at: http://www.ncbi.nlm.nih.gov/pubmed/6836297. Accessed February 2, 2018.
2. Waldorf HA, Kauvar AN, Geronemus RG. Skin resurfacing of fine to deep rhytides using a char-free carbon dioxide laser in 47 patients. Dermatol Surg 1995;21(11):940–6. Available at: http://www.ncbi.nlm.nih.gov/pubmed/7582831. Accessed February 2, 2018.
3. Fitzpatrick RE, Goldman MP, Satur NM, et al. Pulsed carbon dioxide laser resurfacing of photo-aged facial skin. Arch Dermatol 1996;132(4):395–402. Available at: http://www.ncbi.nlm.nih.gov/pubmed/8629842. Accessed January 24, 2018.
4. Alster TS, West TB. Resurfacing of atrophic facial acne scars with a high-energy, pulsed carbon dioxide laser. Dermatol Surg 1996;22(2):151–4. Available at: http://www.ncbi.nlm.nih.gov/pubmed/8608377. Accessed February 2, 2018.
5. Kuo T, Speyer MT, Ries WR, et al. Collagen thermal damage and collagen synthesis after cutaneous laser resurfacing. Lasers Surg Med 1998;23(2):66–71. Available at: http://www.ncbi.nlm.nih.gov/pubmed/9738540. Accessed February 2, 2018.
6. Kelly KM, Majaron B, Nelson JS. Nonablative laser and light rejuvenation: the newest approach to photodamaged skin. Arch Facial Plast Surg 2001; 3(4):230–5. Available at: http://www.ncbi.nlm.nih.gov/pubmed/11710855. Accessed February 2, 2018.

7. Nanni CA, Alster TS. Complications of carbon dioxide laser resurfacing. An evaluation of 500 patients. Dermatol Surg 1998;24(3):315–20. Available at: http://www.ncbi.nlm.nih.gov/pubmed/9537005. Accessed February 2, 2018.

8. Altshuler GB, Anderson RR, Manstein D, et al. Extended theory of selective photothermolysis. Lasers Surg Med 2001;29(5):416–32. Available at: http://www.ncbi.nlm.nih.gov/pubmed/11891730. Accessed February 2, 2018.

9. Ross EV, Mckinlay JR, Sajben FP, et al. Use of a novel erbium laser in a Yucatan minipig: a study of residual thermal damage, ablation, and wound healing as a function of pulse duration. Lasers Surg Med 2002;30:93–100.

10. Manstein D, Herron GS, Sink RK, et al. Fractional photothermolysis: a new concept for cutaneous remodeling using microscopic patterns of thermal injury. Lasers Surg Med 2004;34(34). https://doi.org/10.1002/lsm.20048.

11. Haedersdal M, Sakamoto FH, Farinelli WA, et al. Fractional CO_2 laser-assisted drug delivery. Lasers Surg Med 2010;42(2):113–22.

12. Brightman LA, Brauer JA, Anolik R, et al. Ablative and fractional ablative lasers. Dermatol Clin 2009;27(4):479–89.

13. Geronemus RG. Fractional photothermolysis: current and future applications. Lasers Surg Med 2006;38:169–76.

14. Hunzeker CM, Weiss ET, Geronemus RG. Fractionated CO2 laser resurfacing: our experience with more than 2000 treatments. Aesthet Surg J 2009;29(4):317–22.

15. Alexiades-Armenakas MR, Dover JS, Arndt KA. The spectrum of laser skin resurfacing: nonablative, fractional, and ablative laser resurfacing. J Am Acad Dermatol 2008;58(5):719–37.

16. Shamsaldeen O, Peterson JD, Goldman MP. The adverse events of deep fractional CO2: a retrospective study of 490 treatments in 374 patients. Lasers Surg Med 2011;43(6):453–6.

17. Campbell TM, Goldman MP. Adverse events of fractionated carbon dioxide laser. Dermatol Surg 2010;36(11):1645–50.

18. Fisher GH, Geronemus RG. Short-term side effects of fractional photothermolysis. Dermatol Surg 2005;31(9 Pt 2):1245–9 [discussion: 1249]. Available at: http://www.ncbi.nlm.nih.gov/pubmed/16176779. Accessed February 3, 2018.

19. Na J-I, Choi J-W, Choi H-R, et al. Rapid healing and reduced erythema after ablative fractional carbon dioxide laser resurfacing combined with the application of autologous platelet-rich plasma. Dermatol Surg 2011;37(4):463–8.

20. Lee JW, Kim BJ, Kim MN, et al. The efficacy of autologous platelet rich plasma combined with ablative carbon dioxide fractional resurfacing for acne scars: a simultaneous split-face trial. Dermatol Surg 2011;37(7):931–8.

21. Shin M-K, Lee J-H, Lee S-J, et al. Platelet-rich plasma combined with fractional laser therapy for skin rejuvenation. Dermatol Surg 2012;38(4):623–30.

22. Gawdat HI, Hegazy RA, Fawzy MM, et al. Autologous platelet rich plasma: topical versus intradermal after fractional ablative carbon dioxide laser treatment of atrophic acne scars. Dermatol Surg 2014;40(2):152–61.

23. Kim H, Gallo J. Evaluation of the effect of platelet-rich plasma on recovery after ablative fractional photothermolysis. JAMA Facial Plast Surg 2015;17(2):97–102.

24. Faghihi G, Keyvan S, Asilian A, et al. Efficacy of autologous platelet-rich plasma combined with fractional ablative carbon dioxide resurfacing laser in treatment of facial atrophic acne scars: a split-face randomized clinical trial. Indian J Dermatol Venereol Leprol 2016;82(2):162.

25. Abdel Aal AM, Ibrahim IM, Sami NA, et al. Evaluation of autologous platelet-rich plasma plus ablative carbon dioxide fractional laser in the treatment of acne scars. J Cosmet Laser Ther 2017;0(0):1–8.

26. Hui Q, Chang P, Guo B, et al. The clinical efficacy of autologous platelet-rich plasma combined with ultra-pulsed fractional CO_2 laser therapy for facial rejuvenation. Rejuvenation Res 2017;20(1):25–31.

27. Min S, Yoon JY, Park SY, et al. Combination of platelet rich plasma in fractional carbon dioxide laser treatment increased clinical efficacy of for acne scar by enhancement of collagen production and modulation of laser-induced inflammation. Lasers Surg Med 2017. https://doi.org/10.1002/lsm.22776.

28. Aust MC, Reimers K, Repenning C, et al. Percutaneous collagen induction: minimally invasive skin rejuvenation without risk of hyperpigmentation—fact or fiction? Plast Reconstr Surg 2008;122(5):1553–63.

29. Aust MC, Reimers K, Gohritz A, et al. Percutaneous collagen induction. Scarless skin rejuvenation: fact or fiction? Clin Exp Dermatol 2010;35(4):437–9.

30. Schwarz M, Laaff H. A prospective controlled assessment of microneedling with the dermaroller device. Plast Reconstr Surg 2011;127(6):146e–8e.

31. Aust MC, Knobloch K, Reimers K, et al. Percutaneous collagen induction therapy: an alternative treatment for burn scars. Burns 2010;36(6):836–43.

32. Aust MC, Fernandes D, Kolokythas P, et al. Percutaneous collagen induction therapy: an alternative treatment for scars, wrinkles, and skin laxity. Plast Reconstr Surg 2008;121(4):1421–9.

33. Hou A, Cohen B, Haimovic A, et al. Microneedling: a comprehensive review. Dermatol Surg 2017;43(3):321–39.

34. Iriarte C, Awosika O, Rengifo-Pardo M, et al. Review of applications of microneedling in dermatology. Clin Cosmet Investig Dermatol 2017;10:289–98.

35. Alster TS, Graham PM. Microneedling. Dermatol Surg 2017;1. https://doi.org/10.1097/DSS.0000000000001248.

36. Chawla S. Split face comparative study of microneedling with PRP versus microneedling with vitamin C in treating atrophic post acne scars. J Cutan Aesthet Surg 2014;7(4):209–12.

37. Asif M, Kanodia S, Singh K. Combined autologous platelet-rich plasma with microneedling verses microneedling with distilled water in the treatment of atrophic acne scars: a concurrent split-face study. J Cosmet Dermatol 2016;15(4):434–43.

38. El-Domyati M, Abdel-Wahab H, Hossam A. Microneedling combined with platelet-rich plasma or trichloroacetic acid peeling for management of acne scarring: a split-face clinical and histologic comparison. J Cosmet Dermatol 2017. https://doi.org/10.1111/jocd.12459.

39. Ibrahim MK, Ibrahim SM, Salem AM. Skin microneedling plus platelet-rich plasma versus skin microneedling alone in the treatment of atrophic post acne scars: a split face comparative study. J Dermatolog Treat 2017;1–6. https://doi.org/10.1080/09546634.2017.1365111.

40. Ibrahim ZA, El-Ashmawy AA, Shora OA. Therapeutic effect of microneedling and autologous platelet-rich plasma in the treatment of atrophic scars: a randomized study. J Cosmet Dermatol 2017;16(3):388–99.

41. Frautschi RS, Hashem AM, Halasa B, et al. Current evidence for clinical efficacy of platelet rich plasma in aesthetic surgery: a systematic review. Aesthet Surg J 2017;37(3):353–62.

42. Sand JP, Nabili V, Kochhar A, et al. Platelet-rich plasma for the aesthetic surgeon. Facial Plast Surg 2017;33(4):437–43.

43. Lynch MD, Bashir S. Applications of platelet-rich plasma in dermatology: a critical appraisal of the literature. J Dermatolog Treat 2016;27(3):285–9.

44. Matras H. Die Wirkungen vershiedener Fibrinpraparate auf Kontinuitat-strennungen der Rattenhaut. Osterr Z Stomatol 1970;67:338–59.

45. Weibrich G, Kleis WKG, Hafner G, et al. Growth factor levels in platelet-rich plasma and correlations with donor age, sex, and platelet count. J Craniomaxillofac Surg 2002;30(2):97–102.

46. Marx RE. Platelet-rich plasma: evidence to support its use. J Oral Maxillofac Surg 2004;62(4):489–96.

47. Sundaram H, Mehta RC, Norine JA, et al. Topically applied physiologically balanced growth factors: a new paradigm of skin rejuvenation. J Drugs Dermatol 2009;8(5 Suppl Skin Rejuvenation):4–13. Available at: http://www.ncbi.nlm.nih.gov/pubmed/19562882. Accessed February 2, 2018.

48. Kim DH, Je YJ, Kim CD, et al. Can platelet-rich plasma be used for skin rejuvenation? evaluation of effects of platelet-rich plasma on human dermal fibroblast. Ann Dermatol 2011;23(4):424.

49. Li ZJ, Choi H-I, Choi D-K, et al. Autologous platelet-rich plasma: a potential therapeutic tool for promoting hair growth. Dermatol Surg 2012;38(7pt1):1040–6.

50. Yuksel EP, Sahin G, Aydin F, et al. Evaluation of effects of platelet-rich plasma on human facial skin. J Cosmet Laser Ther 2014;16(5):206–8.

51. Abuaf OK, Yildiz H, Baloglu H, et al. Histologic evidence of new collagen formulation using platelet rich plasma in skin rejuvenation: a prospective controlled clinical study. Ann Dermatol 2016;28(6):718.

52. Fabi S, Sundaram H. The potential of topical and injectable growth factors and cytokines for skin rejuvenation. Facial Plast Surg 2014;30(2):157–71.

53. Martin P. Wound healing: aiming for perfect skin regeneration. Science 1997;276(5309):75–81. Available at: http://www.ncbi.nlm.nih.gov/pubmed/9082989. Accessed February 2, 2018.

54. Fabbrocini G, Annunziata MC, D'Arco V, et al. Acne scars: pathogenesis, classification and treatment. Dermatol Res Pract 2010;2010:893080.

55. Kang S, Cho S, Chung JH, et al. Inflammation and extracellular matrix degradation mediated by activated transcription factors nuclear factor-kappaB and activator protein-1 in inflammatory acne lesions in vivo. Am J Pathol 2005;166(6):1691–9. Available at: http://www.ncbi.nlm.nih.gov/pubmed/15920154. Accessed February 1, 2018.

56. Puizina-Ivić N. Skin aging. Acta Dermatovenerol Alp Pannonica Adriat 2008;17(2):47–54.

57. Fisher GJ, Kang S, Varani J, et al. Mechanisms of photoaging and chronological skin aging. Arch Dermatol 2002;138(11):1462–70. Available at: http://www.ncbi.nlm.nih.gov/pubmed/12437452. Accessed February 1, 2018.

58. Makrantonaki E, Zouboulis CC. Molecular mechanisms of skin aging: state of the art. Ann N Y Acad Sci 2007;1119(1):40–50.

59. Farage MA, Miller KW, Elsner P, et al. Intrinsic and extrinsic factors in skin ageing: a review. Int J Cosmet Sci 2008;30(2):87–95.

60. El-Domyati M, Attia S, Saleh F, et al. Intrinsic aging vs. photoaging: a comparative histopathological, immunohistochemical, and ultrastructural study of skin. Exp Dermatol 2002;11(5):398–405.

61. Mori Y, Hatamochi A, Arakawa M, et al. Reduced expression of mRNA for transforming growth factor beta (TGF beta) and TGF beta receptors I and II and decreased TGF beta binding to the receptors in in vitro-aged fibroblasts. Arch Dermatol Res 1998;290(3):158–62. Available at: http://www.ncbi.nlm.nih.gov/pubmed/9558492. Accessed February 2, 2018.

62. Anitua E. Plasma rich in growth factors: preliminary results of use in the preparation of future sites for implants. Int J Oral Maxillofac Implants 1999;14(4):529–35. Available at: http://www.ncbi.nlm.nih.gov/pubmed/10453668. Accessed November 3, 2017.

63. Gonshor A. Technique for producing platelet-rich plasma and platelet concentrate: background and process. Int J Periodontics Restorative Dent 2002; 22(6):547–57. Available at: http://www.ncbi.nlm.nih.gov/pubmed/12516826. Accessed November 3, 2017.

64. Marx RE, Carlson ER, Eichstaedt RM, et al. Platelet-rich plasma: growth factor enhancement for bone grafts. Oral Surg Oral Med Oral Pathol Oral Radiol Endod 1998;85(6):638–46. Available at: https://ac.els-cdn.com/S1079210498900294/1-s2.0-S1079210498900294-main.pdf?_tid=877bf302-c01c-11e7-98dd-00000aacb360&acdnat=1509661622_a352e18d918c323d2dffa55b26cc0fbe. Accessed November 2, 2017.

65. Dohan Ehrenfest DM, Rasmusson L, Albrektsson T. Classification of platelet concentrates: from pure platelet-rich plasma (P-PRP) to leucocyte- and platelet-rich fibrin (L-PRF). Trends Biotechnol 2009; 27(3):158–67.

66. RE M. Platelet-rich plasma (PRP): what is PRP and what is not PRP? Implant Dent 2001;10(4):225–8. Available at: http://regenmedicalohio.com/wp-content/uploads/sites/58/2014/11/B2-What-is-PRP-Marx-2.pdf. Accessed November 8, 2017.

67. Haynesworth S, Kadiyala S, Liang L. Mitogenic stimulation of human mesenchymal stem cells by platelet releasate suggest a mechanism for enhancement of bone repair by platelet concentrates. Presented at the 48th Annual Meeting of the Orthopaedic Research Society, Dallas, Texas, February 10-13, 2002.

68. Giusti I, Rughetti A, D'Ascenzo S, et al. Identification of an optimal concentration of platelet gel for promoting angiogenesis in human endothelial cells. Transfusion 2009;49(4):771–8.

69. Gawdat HI, Tawdy AM, Hegazy RA, et al. Autologous platelet-rich plasma versus readymade growth factors in skin rejuvenation: a split face study. J Cosmet Dermatol 2017;16(2):258–64.

70. Hu S, Hsiao W-C, Chen M-C, et al. Ablative fractional erbium-doped yttrium aluminum garnet laser with coagulation mode for the treatment of atrophic acne scars in Asian skin. Dermatol Surg 2011;37(7):939–44.

71. Majid I, Imran S. Fractional CO_2 laser resurfacing as monotherapy in the treatment of atrophic facial acne scars. J Cutan Aesthet Surg 2014;7(2):87.

72. Doddaballapur S. Microneedling with dermaroller. J Cutan Aesthet Surg 2009;2(2):110–1.

73. Soltani-Arabshahi R, Wong JW, Duffy KL, et al. Facial allergic granulomatous reaction and systemic hypersensitivity associated with microneedle therapy for skin rejuvenation. JAMA Dermatol 2014;150(1):68.

74. Goodman GJ, Baron JA. Postacne scarring: a qualitative global scarring grading system. Dermatol Surg 2006;32(12):1458–66.

75. Goodman GJ, Baron JA. Postacne scarring–a quantitative global scarring grading system. J Cosmet Dermatol 2006;5(1):48–52.

76. Fabbrocini G, Fardella N, Monfrecola A, et al. Acne scarring treatment using skin needling. Clin Exp Dermatol 2009;34(8):874–9.

77. Magalon J, Bausset O, Serratrice N, et al. Characterization and comparison of 5 platelet-rich plasma preparations in a single-donor model. Arthroscopy 2014;30(5):629–38.

78. Everts PAM, Brown Mahoney C, Hoffmann JJML, et al. Platelet-rich plasma preparation using three devices: implications for platelet activation and platelet growth factor release. Growth Factors 2006;24(3):165–71.

79. Oh JH, Kim W, Park KU, et al. Comparison of the cellular composition and cytokine-release kinetics of various platelet-rich plasma preparations. Am J Sports Med 2015;43(12):3062–70.

80. Castillo TN, Pouliot MA, Kim HJ, et al. Comparison of growth factor and platelet concentration from commercial platelet-rich plasma separation systems. Am J Sports Med 2011;39(2):266–71.

81. Kushida S, Kakudo N, Morimoto N, et al. Platelet and growth factor concentrations in activated platelet-rich plasma: a comparison of seven commercial separation systems. J Artif Organs 2014;17(2):186–92.

Platelet-Rich Plasma for Hair Loss
Review of Methods and Results

Karam W. Badran, MD[a], Jordan P. Sand, MD[b,c],*

KEYWORDS

- Platelet rich plasma • PRP • Androgenetic alopecia • Hair regrowth • Hair regeneration

KEY POINTS

- Hair loss for men and women continues to be a significant problem.
- Traditional treatment strategies have largely been limited to pharmaceutical and surgical modalities.
- PRP for hair restoration is an off-label procedure, as such methods and outcomes reporting are varied within the current literature. Standardization is currently underway through several clinical trials.
- An overall positive clinical response to the use of PRP for hair restoration in androgenetic alopecia and alopecia areata is observed following at least 3 treatments with 4 week intervals between intradermal injections.

INTRODUCTION

Hair loss for men and women continues to be a significant problem worldwide with an estimated volume of more than 600,000 surgical hair restoration procedures performed in 2016 alone.[1] Traditional treatment strategies have largely been limited to pharmaceutical and surgical modalities. Currently approved medications, such as Finasteride and Minoxidil, require a great degree of compliance for long periods of time with varying degrees of effectiveness.[2,3] Side effects are also common and often dissuade use, including sexual dysfunction, mood disorders, increased risks of prostate/breast cancer, and birth defects.[4,5] Surgical treatments, once limited to scalp reduction and rotational flap techniques, have evolved to follicular unit isolation/extraction with the use of punch biopsies or donor strip harvesting. Success and efficiency are affected by surgeon skill set, however, because follicle transection rates and operative speed are limiting factors for both physician and patient.[1,6] In addition, scar, poor wound healing, and an unnatural hairline are frequently reported concerns and considerations in the hands of less experienced surgeons.[7,8] Recent discoveries in the molecular pathways of the hair cycle, however, have provided the foundation for novel investigations in a "biologically oriented" approach to cell-based therapies in hair restoration.[9–12]

The use of platelet concentrates in regenerative medicine has long been investigated in several surgical and clinical fields. The effects of these concentrates on bone grafting and wound healing have been demonstrated in oral and maxillofacial, orthopedic, and cardiac surgery.[13–15] More recently, interest has been increasing in

Disclosure Statement: No financial relationships or disclosures from both authors, K.W. Badran and J.P. Sand.
[a] Department of Head and Neck Surgery, David Geffen School of Medicine, University of California, Los Angeles, 10833 Le Conte Avenue, CHS 62-237, Los Angeles, CA 90095, USA; [b] Spokane Center for Facial Plastic Surgery, 217 West Cataldo Avenue, Spokane, WA 99201, USA; [c] Department of Otolaryngology–Head and Neck Surgery, University of Washington School of Medicine, 1959 NE Pacific Street, Seattle, WA 98195, USA
* Corresponding author. Spokane Center for Facial Plastic Surgery, 217 West Cataldo Avenue, Spokane, WA 99201.
E-mail address: drsand@sandplasticsurgery.com

Facial Plast Surg Clin N Am 26 (2018) 469–485
https://doi.org/10.1016/j.fsc.2018.06.008
1064-7406/18/© 2018 Elsevier Inc. All rights reserved.

dermatology and plastic surgery in both fat grafting and skin rejuvenation.[16–18] Essential to wound repair and the inflammatory/remodeling pathway, platelets contain several chemotactic and mitogenic proteins that are released upon activation; growth hormones and cytokines are among the most prominent biologically active and secreted components.[19,20] Platelet-rich plasma (PRP) is an autogenous, liquid, platelet concentrate that is extracted from a patient's peripheral blood by a centrifugation process. Because PRP is autologous, the risk of hypersensitivity or immunogenic reactions and disease transmission is significantly reduced. The platelet and plasma growth factors isolated in the PRP slurry have been found to be in higher concentration per volume, when compared with a patient's whole blood.[20] The platelet solution may then be activated in vitro (turning to a gelatinous state) or injected in liquid form for activation in vivo.[21,22]

Once activated, platelets release alpha-granules containing a myriad of growth factors, including transforming growth factor-ß (TGF-ß), epidermal growth factor (EGF), basic fibroblast growth factor, vascular endothelial growth factor (VEGF), platelet-derived growth factor (PDGF), and insulin-like growth factor-1 (IGF-1).[19,23,24] These factors have been found to have substantial effects on the hair cell growth cycle: stimulating differentiation proliferation, and hair follicle growth. In brief, the hair cycle consists of a resting telogen phase, an active anagen growing phase, and an apoptotic catagen phase.[25,26] Aberrancies in the cycling of these phases lead to a disruption in hair follicle growth and hair loss. Bulge cells, inducible stem cells found along the shaft of the hair follicle, have been found to repopulate the hair follicle epithelium and are fundamental to the progression of hair cycling.[26,27] It is these hair follicle stem cells that contain growth factor receptors responsible for hair growth

manipulation and molecular pathway regulation.[27] An overview of the growth factor role on hair cell morphogenesis and progression of the hair cycle is provided in **Table 1**. Additional information on the hair cycle can be found within this special issue of *Facial Plastic Surgery Clinics of North America*.

Given the substantial advances in hair cell research, the effects of PRP on hair restoration are promising and have led to several publications over the past decade. With the rapid production of off-label techniques, protocols, and outcomes, a summary of currently used systems and results is informative for all physicians using a biologics approach to hair restoration.

PATIENT EVALUATION, SELECTION, AND CONTRAINDICATIONS
Evaluation

As with the evaluation of all patients concerned with thinning hair, a thorough medical history and physical examination must be performed. A comprehensive approach to the evaluation and diagnosis of the hair loss patient is reported by Mubki and colleagues.[41] Duration, initiation, associated symptoms, present and past medical history, as well as family history aid in differentiating disorders of hair growth, which include androgenetic alopecia (AGA), alopecia areata (AA), anagen/telogen effluvium, cicatricial alopecia, traction alopecia, and other metabolic, infectious, endocrine, or autoimmune disorders. Laboratory tests to aid with diagnosis include complete blood cell count; and measurement of serum levels of iron, serum ferritin, total iron-binding capacity, folic acid, triiodothyronine, thyroxine, thyroid-stimulating hormone, antithyroid peroxidase, dehydroepiandrosterone, testosterone, prolactin, follicle stimulating hormone, and luteinizing hormone.[42,43] Of note, medication history known to affect the cyclooxygenase

Table 1 Growth factors involved in the hair cycle	
TGF-ß	Development of placode and follicular architecture[28]; induction of anagen phase regulated by Tsukushi signaling molecule[29]; regulates endothelial chemotaxis and angiogenesis[30]
FGF	Hair follicle precursor formation[31]; induction and maintenance of anagen from telogen phase via ß-catenin[32]
VEGF	Secreted by dermal papilla cells; promotes angiogenesis and vessel permeability[30]; essential during anagen phase on follicle size[33,34]
PDGF	Development of dermal papilla from epithelium[28] enhances proliferation and is redundant throughout cycle[35–37]
IGF-1	Regulates cell proliferation and migration; prevents catagen phase[38,39]
EGF	Promotes proliferation of outer root sheath hair cells in anagen phase[40]

inflammatory pathway should be documented; these include nonsteroidal anti-inflammatory drugs such as aspirin, glucocorticoids, and immunomodulating therapies.

Selection

The rapid development and increase of investigations into the effects of PRP on hair regeneration have demonstrated positive trends in several studies; however, its off-label use has delayed a robust trial in standardized patient populations. Schiavone and colleagues[44] demonstrated a greater likelihood of subjective improvement in hair growth for patients with moderate (odds ratio 4.1) and severe (odds ratio 7.0) pretreatment global physician assessment scores. Alves and Grimalt[45] found statistically significant correlations in the average total hair density following PRP treatment of AGA in men $\leq$40 years old, with hair loss beginning after the age of 25, and a greater than 10-year evolution of AGA when compared with the placebo group. In a recent patient survey, however, Laird and colleagues found patients $\geq$40 years old were more likely to be satisfied than younger patients; this retrospective survey is limited by recall bias. Other studies note subjectively improved, although not statistically correlated, results in patients with early staged alopecia.[43,46] To date, no guidelines by a physician-led medical society or association exist for the use of PRP on hair growth. As such, most trials reviewed have used PRP in the setting of failed approved medical or surgical therapies in an "off-label" manner.[47] Patient selection, therefore, is largely limited to factors contraindicating the autologous harvest and graft of platelet-rich concentrations. In addition, most studies reviewed (**Table 2**) were performed in patients with AGA of varying scalp sites and severity.

Contraindications

Platelet-rich concentrates require the harvest, processing, and grafting of autologous whole blood components. Therefore, discretionary care before phlebotomy must be exercised. An exhaustive listing of eligibility requirements before phlebotomy is documented by the American Red Cross.[66] Contraindications and exclusion criteria in several studies include coagulation disorders, platelet dysfunction, anticoagulant therapy, thrombocytopenia, hemodynamic instability, local infection at the site of blood harvest or graft injection, hepatitis, and patients who are prone to keloid formation.

PLATELET-RICH PLASMA: PRINCIPLES, SYSTEMS, AND REGULATIONS

The rapid growth and interest in PRP have resulted in the development and commercialization of a wide variety of systems. Fundamental to the mechanism of extraction, various forms of platelet-rich methodologies to enhance wound healing and bone growth have been described: pure platelet-rich plasma (P-PRP), leukocyte and platelet-rich plasma (L-PRP), pure-platelet-rich fibrin, and leukocyte-and platelet-rich fibrin.[22] Owing to the lack of standardized preparation or composition of PRP, there is large variance in the nomenclature used, presence of leukocytes, mode of activation, and overall yield of platelet concentration/growth factor. In general, P-PRP and L-PRP are the injectable solutions used in hair restoration therapy, maintained in liquid form with the use of anticoagulant vials.

Harvesting Platelet-Rich Plasma

The production of platelet concentrates for platelet-rich solutions begins with the harvest of peripheral venous blood. Care is taken to reduce platelet injury/fragmentation because mechanical trauma may result in unintentional activation[67]; these measures include the use of large-bore needles and single needle-stick venipuncture attempts.[21,68] The collected specimen can be centrifuged in 1 or 2 steps depending on the preparation system.[14,68,69] The initial, low-force, centrifugation allows the blood components to separate into 3 weight-dependent layers: (1) a top, supernatant, layer of platelet-poor plasma (PPP); (2) a "buffy coat" (BC) middle layer rich in platelets and containing white blood cells; (3) a bottom, red blood cell (RBC) layer.[15] The second step varies in technique among the numerous protocols, however, in concept is an attempt to discard both the RBC and BC layers. In order to remove these layers, the supernatant PPP and BC layers are harvested following the first centrifugation into a separate test tube. Under high centrifugal force, the platelet-rich layer and plasma supernatant are further separated, improving the precipitant yield of platelets from plasma. The final liquid platelet suspension coined PRP aims to be enriched 4 to 7 times that of whole blood to be considered therapeutically effective, shown to be approximately 1 to 1.5 million platelets per microliter to induce mesenchymal stem cell proliferation.[70,71] Values greater than 1.5 million platelets per microliter have been found to decrease angiogenesis.[72]

472

Table 2
Investigations reviewed, study designs, and results reported

Author, Year	Number of Patients Enrolled (M/F)	Alopecia Type	Activated In-Vitro (Y/N)	Treatment (tx) Interval and Duration	Control Group	Maximum Follow up Duration	Microphotography	Macrophotography	Hair Pull Count	Patient Survey	Histology
Uebel et al,[48] 2006	20/0	AGA Male	Y	Once; with FUE graft	FUE without PRP treatment	7 mo	SSD in increase yield of follicular units per cm² compared with control from baseline	ND	ND	ND	ND
Takikawa et al,[49] 2011	16/10	ND	ND	1 tx/2–3 wk; 5 sessions	Saline	12 wk	Dermascopy: SSD in increase of HC and cross-sectional follicle diameter compared with control from baseline	Digital camera: improved thickness, no independent evaluators	ND	ND	Thickened epithelium, proliferation of collagen, fibroblasts, increased angiogenesis
Betsi et al,[46] 2013	34/8	AGA	ND	5 tx/ND interval; 2 mo	None	3 mo	ND	Reduced hair loss, improved hair volume and quality	Negative in 100% of patients following treatment	Overall patient satisfaction mean rating of 7.0 out of 10.0	ND
Trink et al,[50] 2013	20/25	AA	Y	1 tx/1 mo; 3 sessions	1. Triamcinolone 2. Subcutaneous water injection	12 mo	Dermoscopy: SSD in reduction of dystrophic hairs, improved SALT score, and hair regrowth	SSD in increase of hair growth by 3 evaluators	ND	SSD in burning/itching symptoms compared with baseline	SSD in increase in cell proliferation (Ki-67)
Schiavone et al,[44] 2014	42/22	AGA	N	1 tx/3 mo; 2 sessions	None	6 mo	ND	Jaeshke scale +4 improvement of hair thickness in 40%–55% of patients based on 2-evaluator-assessment of macrophotography compared with baseline	ND	ND	ND
Cervelli et al,[51] 2014	10/0	AGA	Y	1 tx/1 mo; 3 sessions	"Physiologic solution"	12 mo	Phototrichogram: SSD in increase of HC, hair density, terminal hair density, vellus hair density compared with control from baseline	ND	ND	ND	SSD in increase of number of follicles, epidermal thickness, bulge cells, Ki67 + basal keratinocytes, and angiogenesis compared with baseline

Study	M/F	Condition	Randomized	Treatment	Control	Duration	Objective measure	Clinical improvement	Pull test	Patient satisfaction	Other
Gkini et al,[43] 2014	18/2	AGA	Y	1 tx/3 wk + booster at 6 mo; 4 sessions	None	12 mo	Dermoscopy: SSD in increase of hair density compared with baseline, maximum mean density at 6 wk, but SSD at 1 y	Overall improvement in hair density and quality	Negative at 6 wk, increasing to average of 6 hairs at 1 y	Overall mean patient satisfaction of 7.1 out of 10.0	ND
Kang et al,[52] 2014	15/11	AGA	ND	1 tx/3 mo; 2 sessions	Placental extract	6 mo	USB camera magnification: SSD in HC and thickness compared with baseline at 3 mo and 6 mo	ND	ND	ND	ND
Khatu et al,[53] 2014	11/0	AGA Male	Y	1 tx/2 wk; 4 sessions	None	12 wk	TrichoScan: average mean gain of 22 follicular units per cm²	Moderate improvement in hair and volume	Negative pull test in 81% of patient	Overall mean patient satisfaction of 7 out of 10	ND
Sclafani,[54] 2014	9/3	AGA	Y	1 tx/4 wk; 3 sessions	None	6 mo	ND	Hair density index (measured by Hair Check device) approached significance ($P = .06$)	ND	ND	ND
Singh,[55] 2015	20	AA	ND	1 tx/4 wk; 6 sessions	None	12 mo	ND	Relapse in 1 of 20 patients treated	ND	ND	ND
Singhal et al,[56] 2015	8/2	AGA	Y	1 tx/2 wk; 4 sessions	Oral finasteride OR topical minoxidil	12 wk	ND	100% of patients had improved hair volume and coverage on global photography compared with control	65% reduction in number of hairs pulled	ND	ND
Gentile et al,[42] 2015	23/0	AGA	Y	1 tx/1 mo; 3 sessions	"Physiologic solution"	24 mo	TrichoScan: SSD increase in HC, hair density, terminal hair density	ND	ND	ND	SSD in epidermis thickness, number of hair follicles, angiogenesis, Ki67+ bulge cells in basal keratinocytes of epidermis and of hair follicular bulge cells compared with baseline
Alves & Grimalt,[45] 2016	12/13	AGA	Y	1tx/1 mo; 3 sessions	Saline	6 mo	TrichoScan: SSD in HC, density, anagen hairs, telogen hairs, and terminal hair density compared with control from baseline	Clinical improvement from baseline	ND	ND	ND

(continued on next page)

Table 2
(continued)

Author, Year	Number of Patients Enrolled (M/F)	Alopecia Type	Activated In-Vitro (Y/N)	Treatment (tx) Interval and Duration	Control Group	Maximum Follow up Duration	Microphotography	Macrophotography	Hair Pull Count	Patient Survey	Histology
El Taieb et al,[57] 2016	39/51	AA	ND	1 tx/1 mo; 3 sessions	1. Topical 5% Minoxidil 2. Subcutaneous saline placebo	3 mo	Dermoscopy: SSD reduced short vellus hairs, dystrophic hairs, compared with placebo from baseline	SSD in in hair regrowth	ND	ND	ND
Garg,[58] 2016	40/0	AGA	ND	Once; with FUE graft	FUE with intradermal saline injection	6 mo	TrcihoScan: SSD in follicle graft density >75% for PRP group compared with control	ND	ND	ND	ND
Mapar et al,[59] 2016	19/0	AGA Male	Y	1 tx/1 mo; 2 sessions	Saline	24 wk	No SSD in terminal and vellus hairs, no SSD in HC compared with control or baseline	ND	ND	ND	ND
Puig et al,[60] 2016	0/26	AGA Female	N	Once	Saline	26 wk	ND	No SSD in HC or mass	ND	13% claimed substantial improvement, 26% felt heavier hair after treatment	ND
Anitua et al,[61] 2017	13/6	AGA	ND	1 tx/1 mo + booster at 7 mo; 5 sessions	None	12 mo	Trichogram: SSD in increase of hair diameter and density	3 evaluator agreement in clinical improvement from baseline. SSD decrease in distribution of thin hair and increase in thick hair	ND	68% patient satisfaction with global appearance; 79% with noticeable decrease in hair loss, 68% with improvement in hair appearance	SSD in increase of epidermal thickness, proliferative keratinocytes (Ki+ 67), angiogenesis

Study	N	Condition		Treatment	Control	Duration					
Gentile et al,[62] 2017	24/0	AGA Male	Y	1 tx/1 mo; 3 sessions	Saline	12 wk	TrichoScan: SSD in increase of HC and density over control; SSD in improvement when using inactive-PRP than active-PRP	Increased HC, density, and darker pigmentation	ND	ND	ND	Increased number of follicles, Ki67+ keratinocytes, follicular bulge cells, and neovascularization compared with baseline
Jha et al,[63] 2017	20/0	AGA	ND	1 tx/45–60 d; at least 3 sessions	None	12 wk	Dermoscopy: increase in number of vellus and total hairs, and diameter	ND	Negative after treatment in 70% of patients	75% patient satisfaction	ND
Kachhawa et al,[64] 2017	50/0	AGA Male	ND	1 tx/3 wk; 6 sessions	Saline	18 wk	TrichoScan: SSD in increase of thickness and density compared with control from baseline	Improvement in hair thickness and quality	Reduced count in hair pull from baseline	55% reported increase in hair density, 70% reported improvement in hair quality and thickness	ND
Tawfik & Osman,[65] 2017	0/30	AGA Female	Y	1 tx/1 wk; 4 sessions	Saline	7 mo	Folliscope: SSD in increase of hair density and thickness	Improvement in hair volume and quality	Negative in 83% following treatment	High overall patient satisfaction with a mean result rating of 7.0 on a scale of 1–10	ND

Manuscripts reviewed are listed. Study designs and results are summarized.

Abbreviations: F, female; HC, hair count; M, male; N, no; ND, not disclosed; SALT, Severity of Alopecia Tool; Tx, treatment; USB, Universal Serial Bus; Y, yes.

Government Regulations

The US regulatory process for blood products is described in the Food and Drug Administration's (FDA) 21 CFR 127 of the Code of Federal Regulations[73]; this is under the prevue of the FDA's Center for Biologics Evaluation and Research. Currently, PRP is exempt from these regulations, and the administration of PRP is considered a medical procedure.[74] Physicians should use proper discretion when using these devices in an "off-label" manner.[47] PRP devices, subject to regulation via the 510(k) premarket clearance process, need only demonstrate equivalent safety and efficacy as legally marketed devices predicate.[75,76] Under these regulations, as of 2015, more than 40 PRP systems have received FDA clearance.

Manual System

The original PRP processing technique was described by Anitua[69] in 1999 using a single-spin technique. This protocol introduces the common concepts described above in addition to platelet activation by use of a 10% calcium chloride solution. In efforts to increase platelet yield, the 2-step centrifugation procedure was marketed by Curasan and Friadent Schutze.[77,78] The manual protocols have provided the groundwork for several of the commercially available automated systems that have improved reproducibility, work-flow efficiency, and platelet and growth factor yield.[15]

Automated Systems and Kits

The rapid adoption of PRP across several medical specialties has resulted in a 3-fold increase in system valuation since 2009, more than $120 million in 2016 estimates.[79] Using cell-separator and optical reader devices, PRP is processed in a hands-free method to final concentrate. Although significantly improving standardized yields, this pace of commercialization of the several devices on the market has resulted in a wide variety of protocols with differences in the amount of platelet enrichment, presence of leukocytes, erythrocytes, and method of platelet activation. As the composition of PRP is dependent on the technique and device used, the heterogeneity between platelet rich grafts has created a challenging environment when critically evaluating investigative trials across institutions.[19,21,22] Studies comparing the bioactive yields and description of PRP systems are limited despite that most of the performed studies noted the variance in system characteristics as a limiting factor in generalized discussions

on patient outcomes[80–83]; **Table 3** lists devices reported in the studies reviewed for this article. In the most comprehensive comparison of platelet concentrating techniques, Kushida and colleagues[84] evaluated 7 PRP devices, and their yields of platelet, leukocyte, erythrocyte, and growth factor concentrations all varied and consisted of a mixture of L-PRP and P-PRP concentrates.

Centrifugation Systems

Despite the potential for standardization through commercial PRP kits, an independent variable to the yield and efficacy of PRP is the centrifugation systems used to separate whole blood into buffy and supernatant layers. Because platelets are activated by both chemical stimulation and mechanical injury, the disruption that occurs from vibration and temperature shifts is not uniform for all centrifugal devices. In addition, centrifugation protocols vary with PRP system recommendations and practitioner discretion when following open-access methods. The variance observed in 4 commercially available centrifuge systems has recently been characterized, noting significant differences in platelet-rich yield of growth factors, architecture, and the complete damage of entire platelet harvested populations.[67] In order to aid the reviewer in conversion between relative centrifugal force expressed in units of gravity (g and revolutions per minute [rpm]), a formula for conversion based on radius of centrifugation, rotor, and rpm has been developed and further aids in critically analyzing investigative technique.[85] The authors of this study recommend a clear description of manufacturer/open-source protocol and centrifuge modifications.[20,67,69]

PLATELET-RICH PLASMA: GRAFTING AND ADJUVANTS
Methods of Activation

All attempts to maintain platelet stability and prevent degranulation are taken before injection. Anticoagulants utilized to prevent platelet activation include citrate salts, trisodium phosphate, and heparin; though the superiority of these products has yet to be studied. In order to use the mitogenic potential of growth factors for angiogenesis, fibroblast differentiation/proliferation, and collagen synthesis, platelet alpha-granules must be released by platelet activation.

In the presence of exogenously administered calcium chloride/gluconate, or endogenously present thrombin and dermal collagen, 95% of presynthesized growth factors are released within 20 minutes to 1 hour.[15,86] Method of activation is dependent on

Table 3
Platelet-rich plasma processing systems

Author, Year	System, Corporation	Centrifugal Force (g), Speed (rpm), and Duration (min)	Whole Blood Harvested (mL)	Volume Grafted	Platelet Concentrate Relative to Whole Blood
Uebel et al,[48] 2006	Manual	C1: 1000 rpm, 10 C2: 5000 rpm, 10	80	ND	2.5-fold
Takikawa et al,[49] 2011	Manual	C1: 1700 rpm, 15 C2: 3000 rpm, 5	15	3 cc/tx	6.13-fold
Betsi et al,[46] 2013	ACR-C Extra; RegenLab	C1: 1500 g, 5 C2: NA	16	8–12 cc/tx	ND
Trink et al,[50] 2013	Manual	C1: 70 g, 8 C2: NA	36	ND	3- to 5-fold
Schiavone et al,[44] 2014	GPSIII Platelet Separation System; Biomet	ND	60	ND	3.5- to 4-fold
Cervelli et al,[51] 2014	Cascade-Selphyl-Esforax system	C1: 1100 g, 10 C2: NA	18	0.1 cc/cm^2	ND
Gkini et al,[43] 2014	RegenKit BCT-3; RegenLab	C1: 1500 g, 5	16	0.05–0.1 cc/cm^2	5.8-fold
Kang et al,[52] 2014	SmartPReP2; Harvest Technologies Corp	ND	60	0.05–0.1 cc/cm^2	5.9-fold
Khatu et al,[53] 2014	ND	C1:1500 rpm, 6 C2: 2500 rpm, 15	20	2–3 cc/session	
Sclafani,[54] 2014	Selphyl; aesthetic factors	C1: 1100 g, 6 C2: NA	18	0.1 cc/session	ND
Singh,[55] 2015	Manual	ND	25	ND	ND
Singhal et al,[56] 2015	ND	C1: 1500 rpm, 6 C2: 2500 rpm, 15	20	8–12 cc/session	ND
Gentile et al,[42] 2015	Cascade-Selphyl-Esforax system; aesthetic factors	C1: 1100 g, 10 C2: NA	18	0.1 cc/cm^2	ND
Alves & Grimalt,[45] 2016	Manual	C1: 4600 rpm, 8	18	0.15 cc/cm^2	
El Taieb et al,[57] 2016	Manual	C1: 3000 rpm, 10	10	ND	4
Garg,[58] 2016	YCELLBIO PRP kit; Ycellbio Medical	C1: 3200 rpm, 4 C2: 3200 rpm, 1	20	0.2–0.3 cc/cm^2	5- to 7-fold
Mapar et al,[59] 2016	PRP Tubex; Moohan Enterprise	C1: 3000 rpm, 6 C2: 3300 rpm, 3	9	0.24 cc/cm^2	3-fold
Puig et al,[60] 2016	Angel PRP; Cytomedix	ND	60	10 cc/session	2.75- to 3.4-fold
Anitua et al,[61] 2017	Manual	C1: 580 g, 8 C2: NA	18	3–4 cc/session	2-fold
Gentile et al,[62] 2017	CPunT Preparation System; Biomed Device	C1: 1200 rpm, 10 C2: NA	55	0.2 cc/cm^2	ND
	Regen Blood Cell Therapy; RegenLab	ND	24	0.25 cc/cm^2	5-fold
	Arthrex Angel System; Arthrex	ND	120	0.25 cc/cm^2	5-fold

(continued on next page)

Table 3
(continued)

Author, Year	System, Corporation	Centrifugal Force (g), Speed (rpm), and Duration (min)	Whole Blood Harvested (mL)	Volume Grafted	Platelet Concentrate Relative to Whole Blood
Jha et al,[63] 2017	Manual	C1: 160 g, 10 C2: 400 g, 10	15	ND	ND
Kachhawa et al,[64] 2017	Manual	C1: 1200 rpm, 8 C2: 2400 rpm, 4	16	0.1–0.2 cc/cm^2	ND
Tawfik et al,[65] 2017	Manual	C1: 1200 g, 15 C2: 2000 g, 10	10	ND	ND

practitioner preference with only one study to date assessing the impact of activated compared with inactivated PRP in hair restoration.[62] Gentile and colleagues[62] investigated these effects in a half head placebo controlled study administered in 3 treatments over a period of 30 days. Although statistically significant differences (SSD) were found at 6 months in hair growth when comparing experimental to control groups, no SSD was found between activated and inactivated PRP. In addition, no SSD was found in the amount of growth factor produced as assessed by immunosorbent assay. In efforts to boost the endogenous thrombin concentration, iatrogenic cutaneous inflammatory responses have also been attempted by microneedling before PRP with improvements in hair pull test and greater than 75% patient satisfaction in 18 patients on their hair growth.[63] Currently, no consensus has been reached as to which method of activation, exogenous or endogenous, is superior for hair regrowth.[87]

Postprocessing Adjuvants

In an effort to improve clinical outcomes, adjuvants to subcutaneous interfollicular injections have been introduced to the literature through means of individual clinical trials. Schiavone and colleagues[44] used an ultrafiltration device to enhance plasmatic vitronectin and fibronectin concentrations from the PPP layer following centrifugation. Because these proteins have been found to improve wound healing in the extracellular matrix, the investigators hypothesize that growth factor activity will be enhanced in the application of hair regeneration.[88] Their results demonstrate a 41% and 55% clinically important macrophotographic improvement following treatment. However, the protein yield in ultrafiltrate of PPP was not quantified nor was a control group used to aid in assessing the utility of the ultrafiltration technique.[44]

In efforts to enhance angiogenesis in the setting of PRP, Kang and colleagues[52] prepared CD34$^+$ hematopoietic stem cells within a platelet-concentrate solution. Their investigation produced successful outcomes in hair density and count from baseline in both experimental and control (placental extract) groups; all male patients, however, were also prescribed finasteride. Neovascularization with the aid of polymers in PRP has also been studied. Takikawa and colleagues[49] used low-molecular-weight heparin (dalteparin) and protamine water-insoluble microparticles in an effort to prolong the bioactive effects of growth factors following platelet activation at the site of injection.[89] Their results demonstrate significant absorption of growth factors in the setting of microparticles, increased new blood vessel formation on histology, and an SSD in average number of hairs and hair density when compared with the control group. These results are encouraging for future applications of polymer-based approaches to hair regeneration.

Grafting Techniques

Several methods of grafting PRP have been used in the literature. PRP has been applied to all areas of the scalp using subcutaneous or intradermal injection. Injection volumes range from 0.8 to 12 cc with variable dosage frequencies, duration, and surface area covered. Currently, no single method exists for optimal PRP concentration dosing.[90,91]

Adjuvant to Hair Transplantation

Although most of the literature regarding PRP and hair restoration involves the application of subcutaneous or intradermal application of PRP into areas of alopecia, few studies have investigated the response to PRP as an adjuvant to follicular unit extraction (FUE). The first reported adjunct to hair transplantation was performed in a prospective half head controlled study by Uebel and colleagues.[48] Following follicular unit harvest, grafts were soaked in twice-centrifuged PRP for 15 minutes and then activated. PRP-supplemented grafts demonstrated a 15% SSD increase in the yield of follicular unit density when compared with the nonsoaked follicular units grafted in 20 androgenetic male alopecia patients. Recently, the use of PRP as an injectable adjunct at the time of intraoperative follicular unit grafting was performed in a prospective randomized controlled trial.[58] Garg[58] injected nonactivated PRP into 20 androgenetic male alopecia patients at the time of follicular unit grafting. The placebo group received injections of normal saline at the time of hair transplantation. Their results demonstrate greater than 75% graft density at 6 months following FUE in all 20 patients who received PRP compared with only 4 in the non-PRP group. In addition, new hair growth was identified at 8 weeks in 16 patients, and at 4 weeks, the PRP-supplemented group demonstrated greater than 75% graft density in 12 patients compared with none in the non-PRP group, demonstrating faster density, reducing the catagen loss of transplanted hair, and activating dormant follicles in FUE-transplanted patients.

OUTCOMES IN HAIR RESTORATION

Various methods are available for the evaluation of hair loss and growth. Generally, these methods have been devised to aid in identifying and diagnosing the clinicopathologic features associated with different hair-loss disease states. As PRP for hair restoration is an off-label procedure, optimal methods for outcomes reporting have not been established and results have been documented using a wide variety of techniques. In general, these methods are grouped as noninvasive (surveys and photography), semi-invasive (trichogram), and invasive (biopsy) methods.[92] Herein, the authors provide a summary of investigations based on the reported outcomes of 23 original investigations and 3 systematic reviews/meta-analyses, consisting of the largest review of the use of PRP for hair restoration (see **Table 2**).

Patient Surveys

In general, patient perspectives of outcomes following PRP treatment have been positive. An overall mean patient satisfaction of 7.0 out of 10.0 is documented in all studies, which list patient satisfaction as a survey outcome; the range of mean scores listed can be found in **Table 3**.[43,46,53,61,63–65] In addition, 70% to 80% of patients have reported improvement in hair

quality, thickness, and appearance and a decrease in hair loss.[61,64] Only one study (Puig and colleagues) reported low patient-survey improvement rates (13.3% of treatment subjects vs 0% of the placebo subjects); this corresponded with their lack of significant objective clinical improvement in a placebo-controlled trail on the effects of a one-time dose of PRP on Ludwig type II female AGA. The study by Puig and colleagues[60] is the only reported attempt of a single subcutaneous treatment of PRP for hair regrowth.

Pull "Traction" Test

The hair pull test is difficult to validate and standardize owing to the high variation among investigators.[92,93] This semiquantitative test, however, has been used in several studies. All studies reporting a pull test demonstrate reductions in hair loss 3 to 12 months following treatment, with negative pull tests (defined as an average of 3 hairs or less per pull) in 70% to 100% of patients.[46,53,63,65]

Histologic Analysis

Hematoxylin and eosin–stained biopsy results have demonstrated similar data following PRP injection when compared with baseline in AGA and AA patients. Cervelli and colleagues[51] and Gentile and colleagues[42] demonstrated SSD in the increased number follicles, epidermal layer thickness, and bulge cells 2 months after treatment when compared with baseline in AGA. Takikawa and colleagues[49] demonstrated thickened epithelium, proliferation of collagen fibers and fibroblasts, and greater numbers of blood vessels around hair follicles in patients treated with PRP and dalteparin and protamine microparticles at 12 weeks. Long-term, 12-month results were demonstrated by Anitua and colleagues[61] with preservation of increased perifollicular angiogenesis. In addition, immunohistochemistry using Ki67[+] nuclear binding antibodies and anti-C8-144B demonstrates the significant increase from baseline of proliferating cells in the basal layer of the epidermis, outer root sheath, follicular bulge cells, basal keratinocytes, and angiogenesis in AGA and AA patients.[42,50,51,61,62]

Global Macrophotography

Subjective in nature, global macrophotography with the use of digital cameras is the most commonly used technique in evaluating hair regrowth. When taken in standardized patient positions, the paired comparison from baseline allows for reduced recall bias in assessing subjective outcomes following treatment. All studies evaluating macrophotography demonstrated improvement in hair quality, thickness, and hair loss when compared with baseline. In order to standardize evaluator rating, Schiavone and colleagues[44] assessed 576 pretreatment and posttreatment images using a 15-point Jaeschke scale by 2 independent evaluators.[94] Using this clinically validated scale, the evaluator sought to assess the incidence of patients who met the "minimal clinically important difference" in hair regrowth following treatment, predetermined to a score of "+4" defined as "moderately better" following treatment at 6 months. The proportion of patients, out of 42 men and 22 women, who reached this clinically important difference following treatment was 40.6% and 54.7% by the 2 raters, respectively. Their study demonstrates evidence that the treatment induces a clinical advantage for male and female pattern baldness.[44]

Another validated macrophotography tool for AA patients was used by Trink and colleagues[50] in their 22-patient randomized double-blind placebo-controlled half head study. The Severity of Alopecia Tool score representing hair regrowth as a percentage of change from baseline was used by 3 independent and blinded evaluators. Their results demonstrate SSD from baseline and control groups at 2-, 6-, and 12-month follow-up intervals.

Microphotography

Dermoscopy and trichoscopy techniques have allowed for the visualization of high-resolution hair and scalp features at ×20 to ×70 magnification, allowing for assessment of hair density, thickness, and count. Trichogram and scanning software have the additional benefit of characterizing plucked hairs for anagen/telogen features; however, phototrichogram is limited by the need to shave the area of interest, which may be contended by some patients.[92,95] These methods are the most quantitative in identifying outcomes in hair regrowth. Most microphotography outcome studies have resulted in positive results with SSDs in mean hair count, density,[42,43,45,49,51,52,58,61,64,65] follicle cross-sectional diameter, anagen/telogen hairs, dystrophic hair count, and terminal and vellus hair density[42,45,57,63] following PRP treatment when compared with baseline and control groups. Two meta-analyses on AGA have pooled the data of several of these studies.

Gupta and colleagues[90] performed a meta-analysis and systematic review on the quantitative outcomes of PRP on AGA assessed by mean hair density through March 2016. Four studies were identified to have quantifiable data to extract

sufficient measures of treatment success. The group concludes that the pooled data of 60 participants produce moderate support for the effectiveness of PRP in AGA.

Giordano and colleagues[91] expanded their meta-analysis to include secondary outcomes of hair thickness and percentage increase in hair number and follicle cross-section. Five studies involving 117 patients were identified with a positive SSD in pooled analysis showing the difference between treatment and control groups in mean difference of number of hairs per squared centimeter. Hair cross-section measurements also favored the PRP group ($P = .005$). Hair thickness and percentage increase in hair count demonstrated positive trends, although did not reach statistical significance.

Lack of Efficacy

Despite the plethora of studies demonstrating positive outcomes following PRP in hair restoration, 2 studies were identified demonstrating a lack of effect. Mapar and colleagues[59] in a randomized controlled trial of 19 androgenetic male-patterned alopecia patients were injected with 0.24 cc/cm^2 doses of twice-centrifuged and calcium gluconate–activated PRP. Despite a 3-fold increase in the number of platelets in the PRP injected, no SSD was identified from baseline in the mean number of terminal and vellus hairs at 1, 3, and 6 months. Given the heterogeneity in PRP processing and centrifugation, it is difficult to assess with certainty the plausible lack of positive results. However, their study did differ from others in that only 2 treatments were performed with an interval of 1 month, and their patient population consisted of only Norwood class 4 to 6 alopecia with most patients (16 of 17) treated having a duration of baldness of greater than 5 years.

Lack of improvement following PRP was also identified by Puig and colleagues[60] in a double-blind, placebo-controlled female AGA investigation. Hair mass index and hair count in women with Ludwig type II female pattern hair loss did not differ from baseline or placebo-saline injections 26 weeks after a single treatment. Despite a 2.7- to 3.4-fold platelet concentration above whole blood, a single treatment of nonactivated PRP did not result in macrophotographic evidence of hair growth. Of critical importance in this study, only one PRP treatment was delivered without any subsequent injections. Both of these negative studies are useful in that multiple injections are likely needed to obtain a measurable improvement in hair restoration.

Complications and Side Effects

The complication profile in all investigations has been minimal, with side effects at time of injection including erythema, edema, headaches, drowsiness, mild pain, temporary swelling, and scalp sensitivity.[90,96] Although unpublished, anecdotal reports of patients developing alopecia with psoriasiform scalp dermatitis 2 to 6 weeks after being treated with PRP is reported in a 2013 editorial by Antonella Tosti.[97] No reports of bacterial, viral, or mycobacterial infections, folliculitis, panniculitis, hematoma, or seroma formation have been documented following PRP. Of note, patients who received PRP for AA in a single study actually demonstrated an SSD in symptom reduction of burning/itching compared with baseline.[50]

SUMMARY, RECOMMENDATIONS, AND FUTURE DIRECTIONS

An overall positive clinical response to the use of PRP for hair restoration in AGA and AA patients is observed in the literature reviewed. Its effects on hair density, count, and thickness have been demonstrated through multiple trials, with positive effects noted in all studies that used a series of at least 3 treatments. Its use as an adjunct to hair transplantation, as well as potential for use with other adjunct technologies (microparticles, CD34+ cells, microneedling), have the ability to further improve a minimally invasive approach to the care of alopecia patients. Furthermore, when compared with traditional oral/topical treatments, the lack of identifiable complications and convenience of treatment provides a positive outlook for future investigations. To help promote the widespread implementation of PRP for hair loss, standardization of reported techniques and protocols should be elucidated.

Frautschi and colleagues[87] found that a critical limitation of current PRP research is the inaccurate description of PRP composition, dosing, activation, and the use of subjective outcome measures. A suggested set of descriptors organized by the FIT PAAW acronym is suggested to help guide future studies in reporting PRP methodologies. The FIT PAAW classification is composed of the following components: (1) Force of centrifugation; (2) the Iteration or sequence of centrifugation; (3) the Time (duration) of centrifugation; (4) Platelet concentration from baseline of whole blood; (5) Anticoagulant use in PRP processing; (6) the utilization of an Activator and type; and (7) the composition of White blood cells. These technical aspects have been demonstrated to have significant effects on platelet concentration and growth factors present.

The investigators recommend and practice the following based on recently published studies and clinical practice on the use of PRP for hair restoration. Appropriately counseled patients with AGA or AA are treated with at least 3 to 4 intradermal injections of PRP into the scalp, spaced 4 to 5 weeks apart. Following the initial sequence of injections, patients are reevaluated for results. Responders are subsequently given the option to continue injections spaced 4 to 6 months apart for persistent effect. Patients are encouraged to continue their other medical hair restoration treatments during the treatment time (finasteride, minoxidil, and similar). Nonresponders are counseled regarding their result, and further injections are not recommended. However, given the overall low risk of adverse events from all published studies, retreating areas with PRP until clinical evidence of hair regrowth could be a reasonable method of treatment planning, although the maximum number of applications has yet to be established. It is important to note that the use of PRP is not regulated by a government agency, and therefore, judicious clinical judgment is advised.

Standardization of treatment dosing protocols, site/area of injection, and injection technique is an area of future investigation. Additional randomized clinical trials with reproducible methods as well as those contrasting the effects of topical/oral medication for hair regrowth will aid in powering larger cohort analyses with reduced study heterogeneity. Currently, there are 7 active clinical trials evaluating the effect of PRP on AGA and AA.[98] Further evidence for the establishment of PRP for the treatment of AGA or AA provides exciting progress in a field where treatment options are currently limited.

REFERENCES

1. Avram MR, Finney R, Rogers N. Hair transplantation controversies. Dermatol Surg 2017;43(Suppl 2): S158–62.
2. Shin HS, Won CH, Lee SH, et al. Efficacy of 5% minoxidil versus combined 5% minoxidil and 0.01% tretinoin for male pattern hair loss: a randomized, double-blind, comparative clinical trial. Am J Clin Dermatol 2007;8(5):285–90. Available at: http://www.ncbi.nlm.nih.gov/pubmed/17902730. Accessed November 6, 2017.
3. Mella JM, Perret MC, Manzotti M, et al. Efficacy and safety of finasteride therapy for androgenetic alopecia. Arch Dermatol 2010;146(10):1141–50.

4. Shenoy NK, Prabhakar SM. Finasteride and male breast cancer: does the MHRA report show a link? J Cutan Aesthet Surg 2010;3(2):102–5.

5. Traish AM, Mulgaonkar A, Giordano N. The dark side of 5α-reductase inhibitors' therapy: sexual dysfunction, high gleason grade prostate cancer and depression. Korean J Urol 2014;55(6):367.

6. Rousso DE, Kim SW. A review of medical and surgical treatment options for androgenetic alopecia. JAMA Facial Plast Surg 2014;16(6):444.

7. Rose PT, Nusbaum B. Robotic hair restoration. Dermatol Clin 2014;32(1):97–107.

8. Lam SM. Complications in hair restoration. Facial Plast Surg Clin North Am 2013;21(4):675–80.

9. Talavera-Adame D, Newman D, Newman N. Conventional and novel stem cell based therapies for androgenic alopecia. Stem Cells Cloning 2017;10:11–9.

10. Marshall BT, Ingraham CA, Wu X, et al. Future horizons in hair restoration. Facial Plast Surg Clin North Am 2013;21(3):521–8.

11. Falto-Aizpurua L, Choudhary S, Tosti A. Emerging treatments in alopecia. Expert Opin Emerg Drugs 2014;19(4):545–56.

12. Miteva M, Tosti A. Treatment options for alopecia: an update, looking to the future. Expert Opin Pharmacother 2012;13(9):1271–81.

13. Patel AN, Selzman CH, Kumpati GS, et al. Evaluation of autologous platelet rich plasma for cardiac surgery: outcome analysis of 2000 patients. J Cardiothorac Surg 2016;11(1):62.

14. Marx RE, Carlson ER, Eichstaedt RM, et al. Platelet-rich plasma: growth factor enhancement for bone grafts. Oral Surg Oral Med Oral Pathol Oral Radiol Endod 1998;85(6):638–46. Available at: https://ac.els-cdn.com/S1079210498900294/1-s2.0-S10792104989002 94-main.pdf?_tid=877bf302-c01c-11e7-98dd-00000 aacb360&acdnat=1509661622_a352e18d918c323 d2dffa55b26cc0fbe. Accessed November 2, 2017.

15. Dohan Ehrenfest DM, Rasmusson L, Albrektsson T. Classification of platelet concentrates: from pure platelet-rich plasma (P-PRP) to leucocyte- and platelet-rich fibrin (L-PRF). Trends Biotechnol 2009; 27(3):158–67.

16. Sand JP, Nabili V, Kochhar A, et al. Platelet-Rich plasma for the aesthetic surgeon. Facial Plast Surg 2017;33(4):437–43.

17. Lynch MD, Bashir S. Applications of platelet-rich plasma in dermatology: a critical appraisal of the literature. J Dermatolog Treat 2016;27(3):285–9.

18. Eppley BL, Pietrzak WS, Blanton M. Platelet-rich plasma: a review of biology and applications in plastic surgery. Plast Reconstr Surg 2006;118(6): 147e–59e.

19. Weibrich G, Kleis WKG, Hafner G, et al. Growth factor levels in platelet-rich plasma and correlations with donor age, sex, and platelet count. J Craniomaxillofac Surg 2002;30(2):97–102.

20. Marx RE. Platelet-Rich plasma: evidence to support its use. J Oral Maxillofac Surg 2004;62(4):489–96.

21. Dohan Ehrenfest DM, Andia I, Zumstein MA, et al. Classification of platelet concentrates (Platelet-Rich Plasma-PRP, Platelet-Rich Fibrin-PRF) for topical and infiltrative use in orthopedic and sports medicine: current consensus, clinical implications and perspectives. Muscles Ligaments Tendons J 2014; 4(1):3–9.

22. Dohan Ehrenfest DM, Sammartino G, Shibli JA, et al. Guidelines for the publication of articles related to platelet concentrates (Platelet-Rich Plasma - PRP, or Platelet-Rich Fibrin - PRF): the international classification of the POSEIDO. POSEIDO 2013;1(1):17–27.

23. Lubkowska A, Dolegowska B, Banfi G. Growth factor content in PRP and their applicability in medicine. J Biol Regul Homeost Agents 2012;26(2 Suppl 1): 3S–22S. Available at: http://www.ncbi.nlm.nih.gov/pubmed/23648195. Accessed November 2, 2017.

24. Vogt PM, Lehnhardt M, Wagner D, et al. Determination of endogenous growth factors in human wound fluid: temporal presence and profiles of secretion. Plast Reconstr Surg 1998;102(1): 117–23. Available at: http://www.ncbi.nlm.nih.gov/pubmed/9655416. Accessed November 7, 2017.

25. Cotsarelis G, Millar SE. Towards a molecular understanding of hair loss and its treatment. Trends Mol Med 2001;7(7):293–301.

26. Paus R, Cotsarelis G. The biology of hair follicles. N Engl J Med 1999;341(7):491–7.

27. Morris RJ, Liu Y, Marles L, et al. Capturing and profiling adult hair follicle stem cells. Nat Biotechnol 2004;22(4):411–7.

28. McElwee K, Hoffmann R. Growth factors in early hair follicle morphogenesis. Eur J Dermatol 2000;10(5): 341–50. Available at: http://www.ncbi.nlm.nih.gov/pubmed/10882941. Accessed November 7, 2017.

29. Niimori D, Kawano R, Felemban A, et al. Tsukushi controls the hair cycle by regulating TGF-B1 signaling. Dev Biol 2012;372(1):81–7.

30. Dhurat R, Sukesh M. Principles and methods of preparation of platelet-rich plasma: a review and author's perspective. J Cutan Aesthet Surg 2014;7(4):189.

31. Barsh G. Of ancient tales and hairless tails. Nat Genet 1999;22(4):315–6.

32. Lin W, Xiang L-J, Shi H-X, et al. Fibroblast growth factors stimulate hair growth through β-catenin and Shh expression in C57BL/6 mice. Biomed Res Int 2015;2015:730139.

33. Yano K, Brown LF, Detmar M. Control of hair growth and follicle size by VEGF-mediated angiogenesis. J Clin Invest 2001;107(4):409–17.

34. Mecklenburg L, Tobin DJ, Müller-Röver S, et al. Active hair growth (Anagen) is associated with angiogenesis. J Invest Dermatol 2000;114(5): 909–16.

35. Tomita Y, Akiyama M, Shimizu H. PDGF isoforms induce and maintain anagen phase of murine hair follicles. J Dermatol Sci 2006;43(2):105–15.

36. Rezza A, Sennett R, Tanguy M, et al. PDGF signalling in the dermis and in dermal condensates is dispensable for hair follicle induction and formation. Exp Dermatol 2015;24(6):468–70.

37. Kiso M, Hamazaki TS, Itoh M, et al. Synergistic effect of PDGF and FGF2 for cell proliferation and hair inductive activity in murine vibrissal dermal papilla in vitro. J Dermatol Sci 2015; 79(2):110–8.

38. Ahn S-Y, Pi L-Q, Hwang ST, et al. Effect of IGF-I on hair growth is related to the anti-apoptotic effect of IGF-I and up-regulation of PDGF-A and PDGF-B. Ann Dermatol 2012;24(1):26–31.

39. Philpott MP, Sanders DA, Kealey T. Effects of insulin and insulin-like growth factors on cultured human hair follicles: IGF-I at physiologic concentrations is an important regulator of hair follicle growth in vitro. J Invest Dermatol 1994;102(6):857–61. Available at: http://www.ncbi.nlm.nih.gov/pubmed/8006448. Accessed November 2, 2017.

40. Zhang H, Nan W, Wang S, et al. Epidermal growth factor promotes proliferation and migration of follicular outer root sheath cells via Wnt/??-catenin signaling. Cell Physiol Biochem 2016; 39(1):360–70.

41. Mubki T, Rudnicka L, Olszewska M, et al. Evaluation and diagnosis of the hair loss patient. J Am Acad Dermatol 2014;71(3):415.e1-15.

42. Gentile P, Garcovich S, Bielli A, et al. The effect of Platelet-Rich plasma in hair regrowth: a randomized placebo-controlled trial. Stem Cells Transl Med 2015;4(11):1317–23.

43. Gkini MA, Kouskoukis AE, Tripsianis G, et al. Study of platelet-rich plasma injections in the treatment of androgenetic alopecia through an one-year period. J Cutan Aesthet Surg 2014;7(4):213.

44. Schiavone G, Raskovic D, Greco J, et al. Platelet-rich plasma for androgenetic alopecia: a pilot study. Dermatol Surg 2014;40(9):1010–9.

45. Alves R, Grimalt R. Randomized placebo-controlled, double-blind, half-head study to assess the efficacy of platelet-rich plasma on the treatment of androgenetic alopecia. Dermatol Surg 2016; 42(4):491–7.

46. Betsi EE, Germain E, Kalbermatten DF, et al. Platelet-rich plasma injection is effective and safe for the treatment of alopecia. Eur J Plast Surg 2013;36(7):407–12.

47. U.S. Food and Drug Administration. "Off-Label" and investigational use of marketed drugs, biologics, and medical devices - information sheet. Office of the Commissioner. Available at: https://www.fda.gov/RegulatoryInformation/Guidances/ucm126486.htm. Accessed November 7, 2017.

48. Uebel CO, da Silva JB, Cantarelli D, et al. The role of platelet plasma growth factors in male pattern baldness surgery. Plast Reconstr Surg 2006;118(6):1458–66.

49. Takikawa M, Nakamura S, Nakamura S, et al. Enhanced effect of platelet-rich plasma containing a new carrier on hair growth. Dermatol Surg 2011; 37(12):1721–9.

50. Trink A, Sorbellini E, Bezzola P, et al. A randomized, double-blind, placebo- and active-controlled, half-head study to evaluate the effects of platelet-rich plasma on alopecia areata. Br J Dermatol 2013; 169(3):690–4.

51. Cervelli V, Garcovich S, Bielli A, et al. The effect of autologous activated platelet rich plasma (AA-PRP) injection on pattern hair loss: clinical and histomorphometric evaluation. Biomed Res Int 2014; 2014:1–9.

52. Kang JS, Zheng Z, Choi MJ, et al. The effect of CD34+ cell-containing autologous platelet-rich plasma injection on pattern hair loss: a preliminary study. J Eur Acad Dermatol Venereol 2014;28(1): 72–9.

53. Khatu SS, More YE, Gokhale NR, et al. Platelet-rich plasma in androgenic alopecia: myth or an effective tool. J Cutan Aesthet Surg 2014;7(2):107–10.

54. Sclafani AP. Platelet-rich fibrin matrix (PRFM) for androgenetic alopecia. Facial Plast Surg 2014; 30(2):219–24.

55. Singh S. Role of platelet-rich plasma in chronic alopecia areata: our centre experience. Indian J Plast Surg 2015;48(1):57.

56. Singhal P, Agarwal S, Dhot P, et al. Efficacy of platelet-rich plasma in treatment of androgenic alopecia. Asian J Transfus Sci 2015;9(2):159.

57. El Taieb MA, Ibrahim H, Nada EA, et al. Platelets rich plasma versus minoxidil 5% in treatment of alopecia areata: a trichoscopic evaluation. Dermatol Ther 2017;30(1):1–6.

58. Garg S. Outcome of intra-operative injected platelet-rich plasma therapy during follicular unit extraction hair transplant: a prospective randomised study in forty patients. J Cutan Aesthet Surg 2016;9(3):157.

59. Mapar MA, Shahriari S, Haghighizadeh MH. Efficacy of platelet-rich plasma in the treatment of androgenetic (male-patterned) alopecia: a pilot randomized controlled trial. J Cosmet Laser Ther 2016;18(8): 452–5.

60. Puig CJ, Reese R, Peters M. Double-blind, placebo-controlled pilot study on the use of Platelet-Rich plasma in women with female androgenetic alopecia. Dermatol Surg 2016;42(11):1243–7.

61. Anitua E, Pino A, Martinez N, et al. The effect of Plasma Rich in growth factors on pattern hair loss. Dermatol Surg 2017;43(5):658–70.

62. Gentile P, Cole JP, Cole MA, et al. Evaluation of not-activated and activated PRP in hair loss treatment:

role of growth factor and cytokine concentrations obtained by different collection systems. Int J Mol Sci 2017;18(2):1–16.

63. Jha AK, Udayan UK, Roy PK, et al. Original article: Platelet-rich plasma with microneedling in androgenetic alopecia along with dermoscopic pre- and post-treatment evaluation. J Cosmet Dermatol 2017;1–6. https://doi.org/10.1111/jocd.12394.

64. Kachhawa D, Vats G, Sonare D, et al. A Spilt Head Study of Efficacy of Placebo versus Platelet-rich Plasma Injections in the Treatment of Androgenic Alopecia. J Cutan Aesthet Surg 2017;10(2):86–9.

65. Tawfik AA, Osman MAR. The effect of autologous activated platelet-rich plasma injection on female pattern hair loss: a randomized placebo-controlled study. J Cosmet Dermatol 2017. https://doi.org/10.1111/jocd.12357.

66. American Red Cross. Eligibility criteria: alphabetical. Available at: http://www.redcrossblood.org/donating-blood/eligibility-requirements/eligibility-criteria-alphabetical-listing. Accessed November 7, 2017.

67. Dohan Ehrenfest DM, Pinto NR, Pereda A, et al. The impact of the centrifuge characteristics and centrifugation protocols on the cells, growth factors, and fibrin architecture of a leukocyte- and platelet-rich fibrin (L-PRF) clot and membrane. Platelets 2017; 0(0):1–14.

68. Gonshor A. Technique for producing platelet-rich plasma and platelet concentrate: background and process. Int J Periodontics Restorative Dent 2002; 22(6):547–57. Available at: http://www.ncbi.nlm.nih.gov/pubmed/12516826. Accessed November 3, 2017.

69. Anitua E. Plasma rich in growth factors: preliminary results of use in the preparation of future sites for implants. Int J Oral Maxillofac Implants 1999;14(4):529–35. Available at: http://www.ncbi.nlm.nih.gov/pubmed/10453668. Accessed November 3, 2017.

70. RE M. Platelet-rich plasma (PRP): what is PRP and what is not PRP? Implant Dent 2001;10(4):225–8. Available at: http://regenmedicalohio.com/wp-content/uploads/sites/58/2014/11/B2-What-is-PRP-Marx-2.pdf. Accessed November 8, 2017.

71. Haynesworth S, Kadiyala S, Liang L. Mitogenic stimulation of human mesenchymal stem cells by platelet releasate suggest a mechanism for enhancement of bone repair by platelet concentrates. Presented at the 48th Annual Meeting of the Orthopaedic Research Society, Dallas, Texas, February 10-13, 2002.

72. Giusti I, Rughetti A, D'Ascenzo S, et al. Identification of an optimal concentration of platelet gel for promoting angiogenesis in human endothelial cells. Transfusion 2009;49(4):771–8.

73. U.S. Department of Health and Human Services. Human cells, tissues, and cellular and tissue-based products. Available at: https://www.accessdata.fda.gov/scripts/cdrh/cfdocs/cfcfr/CFRSearch.cfm?CFRPart=1271&showFR=1. Accessed November 7, 2017.

74. Beitzel K, Allen D, Apostolakos J, et al. US definitions, current use, and FDA stance on use of platelet-rich plasma in sports medicine. J Knee Surg 2014;28(1):029–34.

75. Anitua E, Prado R, Orive G. Closing regulatory gaps: new ground rules for platelet-rich plasma. Trends Biotechnol 2015;33(9):492–5.

76. Weibrich G, Kleis WKG, Hitzler WE, et al. Comparison of the platelet concentrate collection system with the plasma-rich-in-growth-factors kit to produce platelet-rich plasma: a technical report. Int J Oral Maxillofac Implants 2005;20(1):118–23. Available at: https://www.accessdata.fda.gov/scripts/cdrh/cfdocs/cfCFR/CFRSearch.cfm?fr=807.92. Accessed November 7, 2017.

77. Leitner GC, Gruber R, Neumüller J, et al. Platelet content and growth factor release in platelet-rich plasma: a comparison of four different systems. Vox Sang 2006;91(2):135–9.

78. Weibrich G, Kleis WKG, Hafner G, et al. Comparison of platelet, leukocyte, and growth factor levels in point-of-care platelet-enriched plasma, prepared using a modified Curasan kit, with preparations received from a local blood bank. Clin Oral Implants Res 2003;14(3):357–62.

79. Dhillon RS, Schwarz EM, Maloney MD. Platelet-rich plasma therapy - future or trend? Arthritis Res Ther 2012;14(4):219.

80. Magalon J, Bausset O, Serratrice N, et al. Characterization and comparison of 5 platelet-rich plasma preparations in a single-donor model. Arthroscopy 2014;30(5):629–38.

81. Everts PAM, Brown Mahoney C, Hoffmann JJML, et al. Platelet-rich plasma preparation using three devices: implications for platelet activation and platelet growth factor release. Growth Factors 2006;24(3):165–71.

82. Oh JH, Kim W, Park KU, et al. Comparison of the cellular composition and cytokine-release kinetics of various Platelet-Rich plasma preparations. Am J Sports Med 2015;43(12):3062–70.

83. Castillo TN, Pouliot MA, Kim HJ, et al. Comparison of growth factor and platelet concentration from commercial Platelet-Rich plasma separation systems. Am J Sports Med 2011;39(2):266–71.

84. Kushida S, Kakudo N, Morimoto N, et al. Platelet and growth factor concentrations in activated platelet-rich plasma: a comparison of seven commercial separation systems. J Artif Organs 2014;17(2):186–92.

85. Pierce. Convert between times gravity (×g) and centrifuge rotor speed (RPM). Form ID: TR0040.1. Available at: www.thermo.com/pierce.

86. Cheng M, Wang H, Yoshida R, et al. Platelets and plasma proteins are both required to stimulate collagen gene expression by anterior cruciate ligament cells in three-dimensional culture. Tissue Eng Part A 2010;16(5):1479–89.

87. Frautschi RS, Hashem AM, Halasa B, et al. Current evidence for clinical efficacy of platelet rich plasma in aesthetic surgery: a systematic review. Aesthet Surg J 2017;37(3):353–62.

88. Anitua E, Prado R, Azkargorta M, et al. High-throughput proteomic characterization of plasma rich in growth factors (PRGF-Endoret)-derived fibrin clot interactome. J Tissue Eng Regen Med 2015; 9(11):E1–12.

89. Nakamura S, Kanatani Y, Kishimoto S, et al. Controlled release of FGF-2 using fragmin/protamine microparticles and effect on neovascularization. J Biomed Mater Res A 2009;91A(3):814–23.

90. Gupta AK, Carviel JL. Meta-analysis of efficacy of platelet-rich plasma therapy for androgenetic alopecia. J Dermatolog Treat 2017;28(1):55–8.

91. Giordano S, Romeo M, Lankinen P. Platelet-rich plasma for androgenetic alopecia: does it work? Evidence from meta analysis. J Cosmet Dermatol 2017;16(3):374–81.

92. Dhurat R, Saraogi P. Hair evaluation methods: merits and demerits. Int J Trichology 2009;1(2):108–19.

93. Van Neste MD. Assessment of hair loss: clinical relevance of hair growth evaluation methods. Clin Exp Dermatol 2002;27(5):358–65. Available at: http://www.ncbi.nlm.nih.gov/pubmed/12190635. Accessed November 10, 2017.

94. Jaeschke R, Singer J, Guyatt GH. Measurement of health status. Ascertaining the minimal clinically important difference. Control Clin Trials 1989;10(4): 407–15. Available at: http://www.ncbi.nlm.nih.gov/pubmed/2691207.

95. Galliker NA, Trüeb RM. Value of trichoscopy versus trichogram for diagnosis of female androgenetic alopecia. Int J Trichology 2012;4(1):19–22.

96. Laird ME, Lo Sicco KI, Reed ML, et al. Platelet-Rich plasma for the treatment of female pattern hair loss: a patient survey. Dermatol Surg 2017;1–3. https://doi.org/10.1097/DSS.0000000000001109.

97. Valente Duarte de Sousa IC, Tosti A. New investigational drugs for androgenetic alopecia. Expert Opin Investig Drugs 2013;22(5):573–89.

98. Search of: alopecia platelet | Recruiting ClinicalTrials.gov. Available at: https://www.clinicaltrials.gov/ct2/results?term=alopecia+platelet&Search=Apply&recrs=b&recrs=a&recrs=f&recrs=d&age_v=&gndr=&type=&rslt=. Accessed November 13, 2017.

Mesothelial Stem Cells and Stromal Vascular Fraction
Use in Functional Disorders, Wound Healing, Fat Transfer, and Other Conditions

Greg Chernoff, BSc, MD, FRCS(C)[a,b,c,*], Nathan Bryan, PhD[d], Andrea M. Park, MD[e]

KEYWORDS

• Stromal vascular fraction • Adipose-derived stem cells • Nitric oxide • Cellular therapy

KEY POINTS

• Autologous stromal vascular fraction can be released enzymatically from lipoaspirate harvested under a local anesthetic; this is currently not a procedure approved by the US Food and Drug Administration.
• Stromal vascular fraction contains a heterogeneous population of cells, including adipose-derived stem cells, hematopoietic stem cells, endothelial progenitor cells, macrophages, red blood cells, platelets, growth factors, and T-regulatory cells.
• With proper homing and activation events, stromal vascular fraction possesses several key properties, including regenerative, antiinflammatory, immunomodulatory, and pain mitigation.
• Multiple conditions have been treated with stromal vascular fraction, including osteoarthritis, musculoskeletal disease, neurodegenerative disorders, and autoimmune conditions.
• With ongoing research, safety data should continue to be recorded, as well as symptom improvement data, which will continue to validate this form of regenerative therapy.

INTRODUCTION

The ability to regenerate or heal damaged tissue was once considered science fiction, but now autologous fat-derived mesenchymal stem cells is opening new frontiers for patients, particularly those with degenerative, inflammatory, and autoimmune conditions. With the soaring costs of health care, the development of autologous cellular therapies using cells isolated from the human body with cost-effective, safe, sterile, and reliable surgical procedures and tissue transfer techniques could help to dramatically decrease the costs of health care by enabling the science in our bodies to recuperate itself.[1] Additionally, having a supply of one's own cells on demand may also change how accidents, myocardial infarcts, strokes, concussions, paralysis, or sudden

Disclosures: None.
[a] Chernoff Cosmetic Surgeons, Private Practice, 9002 N Meridian Street, Suite 205, Indianapolis, IN 46260, USA; [b] Chernoff Cosmetic Surgeons, Private Practice, 1701 4th Street, Suite 100, Santa Rosa, CA 95404, USA; [c] Chernoff Cosmetic Surgeons, Private Practice, 17 Wenjiing Road, Weiyang, Xian 710032, China; [d] Department of Molecular and Human Genetics, Baylor College of Medicine, 1 Baylor Plaza, Houston, TX 77030, USA; [e] UCLA Department of Otolaryngology Head and Neck Surgery, Facial Plastic Surgery, 200 UCLA Medical Plaza, Suite 500, Los Angeles, CA 90095, USA
* Corresponding author. Chernoff Cosmetic Surgeons, Private Practice, 9002 N Meridian Street, Suite 205, Indianapolis, IN 46260.
E-mail address: greg@drchernoff.com

Facial Plast Surg Clin N Am 26 (2018) 487–501
https://doi.org/10.1016/j.fsc.2018.06.009

illness are treated. The ability to use mesenchymal stems cells in the treatment of carcinoma also exists. Stem cells possess the ability to home in on cancerous tissue. The stem cells can partner with the small pox virus and chemotherapy drugs to selectively attack cancer primaries and metastases, leaving healthy tissue unaffected. Further applications include treatment of acne, alopecia, psoriasis, eczema, sinusitis, healing wounds and wound beds, burns, hypertrophic scars, and keloids. This article provides an overview of mesothelial stem cells and stromal vascular fractionation; however, owing to the cutting-edge nature of these methods, they are not currently approved by the US Food and Drug Administration for use in the United States.[2]

THE SCIENCE OF MESENCHYMAL STEM CELLS

Mesenchymal stem cells possess self-renewal and multilineage differentiation potentials, which makes them an attractive source of stem cells for tissue engineering. Because these mesenchymal cells can be grown and multiplied, they effectively provide one with a long-term supply of a person's own stem cells for treating multiple conditions. Comparative analyses of various sources of mesenchymal stem cells, such as from bone marrow, adipose tissue, umbilical cord, and placental blood, have been done and many evidence-based articles suggest that MSCs have a potentially therapeutic use in the treatment of degenerative, inflammatory, and autoimmune conditions, and in scar mitigation.[3–10] In addition to treating diseases, Song and colleagues[11] demonstrated that injected MSCs activated the Wnt signaling cascade to alleviate pain. Adipose-derived stem cells have also demonstrated the ability to differentiate into many other cells and tissues, other than mesenchymal lines. In veterinary medicine, adipose-derived stem cells have been used to effect chondrogenesis and for other orthopedic conditions. Currently, the most common joints treated with success, include the knees, hips, shoulders, backs, ankles, elbows, fingers, feet, thumbs, and wrists.

THE SCIENCE OF STROMAL VASCULAR FRACTIONATION

Stromal vascular fraction (SVF) can be isolated from subcutaneous fat, and is known to contain adult mesenchymal stem cells, endothelial precursor cells, preadipocytes, antiinflammatory macrophages, T-regulatory cells, and cytokine growth factors.[12,13] Early veterinary experience with SVF explored its safety and efficacy, whereas various other studies highlighted SVF's immunomodulatory capabilities.[14,15] Recently, Guo and Nguyen and their colleagues reviewed the concepts, safety, and efficacy of SVF to date.[16,17] Subsequent research has yielded innovative methods of cryogenically freezing SVF so as to provide multiple deployments, both economically and conveniently (Cells on Ice; American Cryostem Corporation, Eatontown, NJ). Despite all that has been published, there are few articles in the literature that specifically looked at therapeutic outcomes. Drs Mark Berman and Elliot Lander initiated The Cell Surgical Network to address this knowledge deficit and fostered a multidisciplinary approach to exploring the potential efficacy of SVF in treating multiple diseases (Cell Surgical Network Data Base, Unpublished Data).[18] Their database includes safety study results on 2000 patients, with a 0.05% complication rate, as well as results from more than 400 physicians working in more than 100 clinics around the world who have treated more than 4000 patients. **Box 1** lists the current institutional review board–approved areas of research within the Cell Surgical Network.

The major cellular components of SVF along with their most defining cell surface markers are listed in **Table 1**. When examined under flow cytometry, no 2 patients' SVF is identical in composition. As shown, the main properties of SVF are antiinflammatory, regenerative, and immunomodulatory. The stem cells deploy to a site that is secreting signaling molecules associated with degenerated, damaged, or inflamed tissue via a process referred to as *homing*. The second essential event in a stem cell operation is *activation*, wherein the stem cells must be effectively turned on by other signaling molecules that are associated with degeneration, damage, or inflammation to effect healing. The antiinflammatory property of SVF explains the pain relief that arthritis and other inflammatory condition patients typically describe, often within 48 to 72 hours of deployment. The second SVF property is its *regenerative potential*, which typically takes several months to occur. With this process, cells are capable of promoting healing by directly replacing damaged cells or secreting cytokine growth factors that affect cellular repair. Last is SVF's ability to be *immunomodulatory*. This capability allows SVF to effectively reset the immune system to correct the malfunction. The main properties of SVF after homing and activation criteria are met include antiinflammatory, regenerative, immunomodulatory, scar mitigation, and pain reduction. Several common problems and disease states affecting the patient undergoing

Box 1
Current conditions treated: institutional review board protocol

Orthopedics
  Neck arthritis and spine disease
  Back arthritis and spine disease
  Knee problems
  Hip problems
  Elbow and hand problems
  Shoulder problems
Neurology
  Multiple sclerosis
  Peripheral neuropathy
  Amyotrophic lateral sclerosis
  Parkinson disease
  Muscular dystrophy
  Stroke
  Incomplete spinal cord injury
Cardiac/pulmonary
  Asthma
  Post myocardial infarction
  Congestive heart failure
  Cardiomyopathy
  Asthma degenerative disease
  Lung disease
Ophthalmology
  Dry eyes
  Macular degeneration
  Glaucoma
  Optic neuritis
  Diabetes-related eye disease
Urology
  Interstitial cystitis
  Peyronie's disease
  Erectile dysfunction
  Male incontinence
Autoimmune
  Lupus
  Relapsing polychondritis
  Autoimmune hepatitis
  Crohn's disease
  Rheumatoid arthritis
  Myasthenia gravis
  Lichen sclerosus

Cosmetic

Fat transfer

Alopecia areata

Dermal atrophy

Acne vulgaris

Data from Berman M, Lander E. A prospective safety study of autologous adipose-derived stromal vascular fraction using a specialized surgical processing system. Am J Cosm Surg 2017;32(3):129–42.

facial plastic surgery should in theory, then, be helped with SVF.

STROMAL VASCULAR FRACTION ISOLATION AND DEPLOYMENT TECHNIQUE

Box 2 details our protocol for isolating SVF. It is then deployed in various manners depending on the condition being treated. The most common routes for deployment are via the intravenous (IV), intraarticular, soft tissue, intrathecal, Omaya Shunt, intraperitoneal, and nebulized routes.

MAXIMIZING STROMAL VASCULAR FRACTION DEPLOYMENT: THE ROLE OF NITRIC OXIDE

Nitric oxide (NO) may be one of the key players in the stem cell regenerative medicine world.

Table 1
Cells in stromal vascular fraction

Cell	Marker
ADSC	$CD45^{low}$
	CD34+
	CD31−
	CD90+
HSC	CD45+
	$CD34^{low}$
	CD14+
	CD31−
	CD206+
M1 macrophage	CD45+
	CD34−
	CD14+
	CD206−
Pericytes	CD45−
	CD34−
	CD146+
	CD31−

Data from Harman R, Cowles B, Orava C, et al. A retrospective review of 60 cases of joint injury in sport horses treated with adipose derived stem and regenerative cell therapy. Vet Stem Biopharma 2016. Available at: https://www.vet-stem.com/pdfs/7605-0003-001%20Equine%20Joint%20Retrospective%20Review.pdf.

NO is a multifunctional signaling molecule, intricately involved with maintaining a host of physiologic processes including, but not limited to, host defense, neuronal communication, and the

Box 2
Stromal vascular fraction deployment technique

After informed consent of procedure and ethical information that the procedure is not approved by the US Food and Drug Administration (FDA), a patient is prepped and draped in appropriate fashion for liposuction. Local anesthetic is infused consisting of 0.5% lidocaine with 1:400,000 epinephrine and 8.4% sodium bicarbonate. A subdermal, nontumescent method of blocking small regions of torso skin is used. Most commonly, the abdomen or flanks are targeted. The Medikan Lipo-Kit system (Medikan International, Inc, Seoul, Korea) is used to harvest, centrifuge, incubate, and isolate the stromal vascular fraction (SVF) (510K approved for fat grafting).

Through a number 11 blade puncture, liposuction is performed. The negative pressure syringe technique is used with a TP-101 syringe and a 3-mm canula. We obtain 50 to 100 mL of lipoaspirate solution and condense it via centrifugation at 2800 rpm for 3 minutes. We add 12.5 Wunsch units of Good Manufacturing Practices grade collagenase (Liberase, Roche, Indianapolis, IN) in 25 mL of normal saline to 25 mL of condensed fat and incubated at 38°C for 30 minutes to digest the collagen matrix to procure the SVF in closed syringes (TP-102 syringe by MediKan) in the operating room.

The product is washed with D5LR sequentially (3 times). This brings collagenase detectable levels to zero. The SVF concentrate is subsequently isolated. The SVF is filtered through an FDA-approved 100 micron nylon filter (BD Falcon cell strainer, Becton Dickinson, Inc, Franklin Lake, NJ). Photomicrography using the Countess Invitrogen (Thermo Fisher Scientific, Waltham, MA) is used to document lack of aggregation, allow a cell count, and measure cell viability using 0.4% trypan blue. Cell viability of SVF, measured by the Countess, typically demonstrated 65% to 95%.

regulation of vascular tone. The primary target of NO is the enzyme soluble guanylyl cyclase that, when activated, leads to the conversion of guanosine 5'-triphosphate to cyclic guanosine monophosphate.[19,20] It is through cyclic guanosine monophosphate that NO is thought to elicit its cell signaling events. It has also been proposed that S-nitrosothiols mediate the actions of NO synthase (NOS) whereby modification of critical cysteine residues by NO or NO-related species modulate protein structure and function, akin to phosphorylation.[21,22]

Endogenous production of NO is a highly complex and regulated process involving the 5-electron oxidation of L-arginine, requiring numerous substrates and cofactors. It is synthesized by enzymes called NOS, such as NOS-1 (neuronal NOS), NOS-2 (inducible NOS), and NOS-3 (endothelial NOS), which catalyzes the oxidation of L-arginine into L-citrulline with the release of NO.[23] This enzymatic NO synthesis from NOS is critically influenced by various cofactors such as tetrahydrobiopterin, flavin mononucleotide, flavin adenine dinucleotide, the presence of reduced thiols, the endogenous NOS inhibitor asymmetric dimethylarginine, and substrate and oxygen availability.[24] Without an adequate delivery of substrate and cofactors (conditions that exist during ischemia), NOS no longer produces NO, but instead transfers the free electrons to oxygen, thereby producing oxygen free radicals.[25] Another production pathway for NO production is through the nitrate–nitrite–NO pathway, whereby inorganic nitrate from the diet is reduced to nitrite and NO by oral nitrate-reducing bacteria.[26,27] Dietary nitrate is an important source of NO in mammals. Green, leafy vegetables and some root vegetables (such as beetroot) have high concentrations of nitrate. When eaten and absorbed into the bloodstream, nitrate is concentrated in saliva (about 10-fold) and is reduced to nitrite on the surface of the tongue by a biofilm of commensal facultative anaerobic bacteria.[28] This is a very important reason for avoiding mouthwashes because they may kill the very bacteria that is designed to keep you healthy by their NO production. The nitrite produced by the oral bacteria is swallowed and reacts with acid, reducing substances in the stomach to generate NO gas. Many lifestyle and dietary habits that lead to chronic disease are linked to insufficient NO. These lifestyle changes are lack of exercise, a poor diet, and some of the medicines that we are prescribed for certain medical conditions, such as antibiotics and antacids.

The production of a highly reactive and diffusible free radical gas to activate a cellular target is a new paradigm in cell signaling and is unique compared with our established concept and model of specific and targeted receptor–ligand interaction to elicit cell signaling events. NO has an effect on almost everything from maintaining blood pressure to preventing many disease conditions to dramatically stimulating stem cells to help heal the human body. NO has been referred to as the Holy Grail of stem cell therapy and is required for stem cell mobilization and differentiation.[29,30] In fact, the bioavailability of NO production in individual patients may predict the success or failure of stem cell treatment. Cell signaling is very important in the field of stem cell science because it is the intercellular communication system of the body. It is how our body tells its own resident stem cells to mobilize and differentiate to repair dysfunctional cells and tissues. Interestingly, our immune system depends on NO production. It is produced by our immune cells and binds to iron sulfur centers within bacteria and other pathogens to shut down their respiration, thereby killing off infectious agents and even tumors. To regulate immune responses, NO triggers the eradication of pathogens on the one hand and, on the other hand, modulates immunosuppression during tissue restoration and wound healing processes. Mesenchymal stem cells are immune modulators, and NO works hand in hand with mesenchymal stem cells and macrophages to make the stem cell environment more conducive for stem cell repair. There is essentially no pathologic condition in the body where NO does not play a role in the management of the condition. Most of the aspects of cell signaling involves cytokines. Their release has an effect on the behavior of the cells around them. Cytokines work as immunomodulation agents. Cytokines include, among other things, chemokines and interleukins, all of which are growth factors typically produced by stem cells, platelets, and various immune cells. One important example of how NO works in signaling involves the concept of hyperbaric oxygen. It has been a long-standing principle that hyperbaric oxygen can increase healing, especially for chronic wounds. However, the mechanism of action of hyperbaric oxygen is through the production of NO rather than increased oxygen.[31]

The inability to produce NO is the earliest event in the onset and progression of most if not all chronic diseases, including cardiovascular disease, the number one killer of men and women worldwide. The problem is that, as we age, we lose our ability to produce NO, so our bodies own ability to heal itself becomes compromised.[32–34] When our ability to produce NO diminishes, we become susceptible to a host of chronic diseases. By the age of 40, most adults produce only about 50% of the NO produced when they were 20. We now know that diminished NO production is a very early marker of chronic disease. The loss of NO generation as a result of a dysfunctional vascular endothelium is a very likely cause of heart disease as well as many if not all other chronic diseases.[35] Continuous generation of NO is essential for the integrity of the cardiovascular system, because decreased production and/or bioavailability of NO is central to the development of cardiovascular disorders.[36,37] NO possesses a number of physiologic properties that make it a potent cytoprotective signaling molecule; these include vasodilation and the inhibition of oxidative stress, platelet aggregation, leukocyte chemotaxis, and apoptosis.[38–40]

Harnessing the power of the cells is the fundamental basis of stem cell regenerative medicine and the key to doing so is through the regulation of NO. NO is a fundamental cellular signaling molecule responsible for a host of physiologic functions and, although it was originally discovered for its effect in maintaining normal blood pressure and cardiac function, NO is now recognized as the requisite signal for stem cell mobilization and differentiation into target cell types.[29,30] The bioavailability of NO in patients may predict stem cell therapy success or failure. Trials using stem cells in patients after infarction have shown highly variable results. This finding can be partly explained by the age-dependent loss of NO production and the inherent NO niche of individual stem cells harvested for injection and treatment. Treating patients or harvested stem cells with NO before treatment may improve the success of stem cell therapy. For optimal success for stem cell therapy, it is important to normalize NO production in patients, especially in patients receiving SVF. This therapy involves different cells in the mixture, including stem cells and endothelial cells. Making the cells more functional by normalizing their NO production improves the efficacy of the stem cell treatment once deployed back into the patient. One way to do this is through the use of a patented NO lozenge, Neo40 (human[n], Austin, TX). Peer-reviewed, published, placebo-controlled studies demonstrate that the NO lozenge could modify cardiovascular risk factors in patients over the age of 40, significantly reduce triglycerides, and reduce blood

pressure.[41] This same lozenge was used in a pediatric patient with argininosuccinic aciduria and resulted in a significant decrease in his blood pressure, as well as reversal of his heart disease and renal disease when other prescription medications proved ineffective.[42] A more recent clinical trial using the nitrite lozenge reveals that a single lozenge can significantly reduce blood pressure, dilate blood vessels, and improve endothelial function and arterial compliance in hypertensive patients.[43] Furthermore, an ongoing study of prehypertensive patients (a blood pressure of >120/80 but <139/89 mm Hg) demonstrated that administration of 1 lozenge twice daily lead to a significant decrease in blood pressure (12 mm Hg systolic and 6 mm Hg diastolic) after 30 days.[44] The same lozenge was used in an exercise study and was found to lead to a significant improvement in exercise performance.[45] Six months use of the NO lozenge led to a statistically 11% significant decrease in carotid plaque.[46] These studies clearly demonstrate the safety and efficacy of restoring NO production in humans and provides a means to restore NO production in patients before and after stem cell therapy. Understanding the role of NO in stem cell biology will help to improve stem cell therapy and reveal novel strategies to replete NO in patients before stem cell harvest and/or treatment of cell before injection to optimize regenerative or healing outcomes.

STROMAL VASCULAR FRACTION AND ACNE

With regard to inflammatory conditions, acne vulgaris and subsequent sequalae can result in a negative impact on a patients' self-esteem. Acne vulgaris is a chronic inflammatory disease that affects 40 to 50 million Americans per year, and hundreds of millions of patients worldwide per year.[47] patients with acne present an excellent model for studying scar pathophysiology. The complex interactions of infection, inflammation, tissue injury, wound healing, and the propensity for scar formation allow scientists a unique opportunity to investigate alternate forms of therapy. Acne is characterized by comedones, pustules, and papules. Left untreated, saucerized and pitted scars can form. The pathogenesis of acne is multifactorial, but 4 primary factors play a pivotal role in the formation of acne lesions: excess sebum production, abnormal keratinization, inflammation, and bacterial colonization of Propionibacterium acnes in the pilosebaceous unit. Although a general consensus exists on the pathogenetic factors,

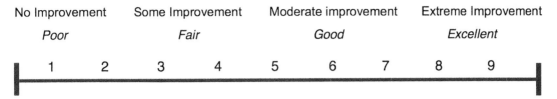

No Improvement	Some Improvement	Moderate improvement	Extreme Improvement
Poor	Fair	Good	Excellent

1   2   3   4   5   6   7   8   9

Fig. 1. Linear analog scale. (*Courtesy of* W.G. Chernoff, Indianapolis, IN.)

the developmental sequence of events has been controversial. A traditional belief was that abnormal keratinization results in the microcomedone, the earliest subclinical acne lesion. Sebaceous gland activation by androgens led to excess sebum production, with a keratin plug being formed. P acnes colonization induced the innate immune system, culminating in the visible inflammation.[48] Although androgen-induced sebum production, follicular hyperkeritanization, and plugging were cited as initial events altering the pilosebaceous unit favoring P acnes proliferation, new evidence suggests a reversal of this order. It is now felt that subclinical inflammation is the inciting factor. Studies have shown significant inflammatory factors surrounding the pilosebaceous unit in clinically uninvolved skin units in patients with acne.[49] Recent data suggest that recognition of microbes such as P acnes triggers an innate immune response via activation of Toll-like receptor 2 (TLR-2), and the inflammasome, a caspase 1–activating cytoplasmic complex that induces the secretion of crucial proinflammatory cytokines.[50] The innate immune system is the body's first line of defense against pathogen-associated molecular patterns and damage-associated molecular patterns. These pathways combat infection and prevent foreign invasion, and also result in tissue inflammation and injury. It is now felt that subclinical inflammation precedes microcomedone formation. Immunohistochemical studies show significant inflammation around normal follicles of uninvolved skin of patients with acne before follicular hyperkeritanization. Another study showed inflammatory cell infiltrates without clinically visible inflammatory lesions. This is thought to be via the proinflammatory cytokine IL-1alpha, independent of colonization.[51]

P acnes induced inflammation has been shown to be mediated by proinflammatory cytokines tumor necrosis factor-alpha, IL-1, IL6, IL-8, and IL-12. P acnes activates the NLRP3 inflammasome which causes monocytes to upregulate caspase 1, an inflammatory caspase required for the proteolytic cleavage, and subsequent

triggering of IL-1beta.[52] IL-8 promotes a T1 response, whereas IL-12 promotes neutrophil chemotaxis, via TLR-2 signaling, which requires extracellular recognition of pathogens. Inflammasome-mediated activation requires internalization and access of the bacterium to the interior compartments of the cell. Therefore, P acnes activates both extracellular (TLR-2 activation), and intracellular triggers of the innate immune response. This finding suggests that P acnes–induced inflammation can be selectively targeted by agents directed at the inflammasome components, IL-1beta, or the TLR-1. These data signify a paradigm shift in the pathophysiology and treatment of patients with acne. All acne is truly inflammatory. By identifying aberrations in a patients' immune response, we can develop targeted treatments for this chronic debilitating disease. To that end, therapies designed to decrease subclinical inflammation should also have benefit.

Given this science, SVF should in theory show benefit for patients with acne. Before initiating patients within the CSN Data Base, proof of concept therapy was undertaken in 4 patients who were treated pro bono. These 4 patients were treated with the CSN protocols, one with IV infusion alone, one with intradermal injection, and two with both IV and intradermal injection. In all cases, acne improved as shown by linear analog tests (**Fig. 1**) for measured features. All patients showed objective acne count improvement (**Figs. 2–5**).

Stromal Vascular Fraction and Other Chronic Conditions

General wound healing should also be facilitated with SVF. Two patients with chronic sinusitis had SVF deployed locally and intravenously at the time of endoscopic sinus surgery. Both patients had more than 5 years of recurrent disease with more than 6 episodes per year and previous surgeries. At the time of this publication, it was too early to determine if the SVF made a statistically significant difference for either of these patients. Anecdotally, both described subjective

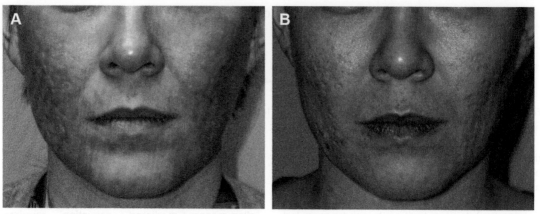

Fig. 2. Acne. (*A*) Study patient before treatment. (*B*) The same patient 4 weeks after intravenous infusion of stromal vascular fraction alone. (*Courtesy of* W.G. Chernoff, Indianapolis, IN.)

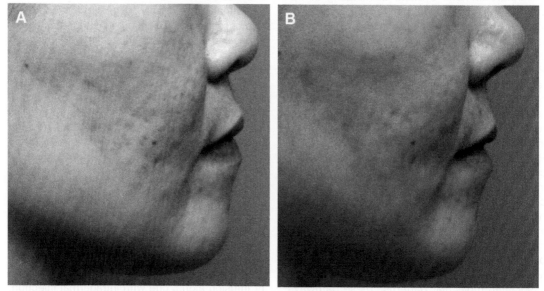

Fig. 3. Acne. (*A*) Study patient before treatment. (*B*) The same patients 4 weeks after intradermal injection of stromal vascular fraction. (*Courtesy of* W.G. Chernoff, Indianapolis, IN.)

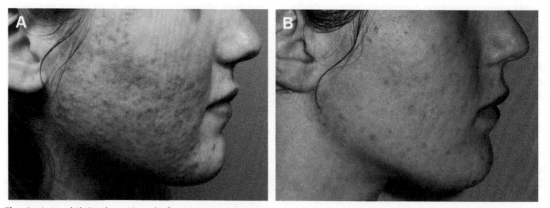

Fig. 4. Acne. (*A*) Study patient before treatment. (*B*) The same patients 4 weeks after intravenous infusion and intradermal injection of stromal vascular fraction. (*Courtesy of* W.G. Chernoff, Indianapolis, IN.)

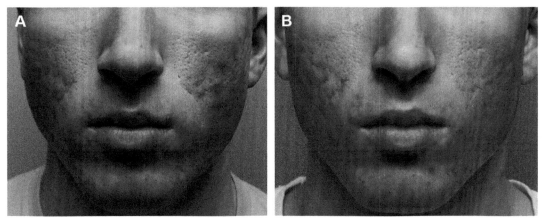

Fig. 5. Acne. (*A*) Study patient before treatment. (*B*) The same patients 4 weeks after intravenous infusion and intradermal injection of stromal vascular fraction. (*Courtesy of* W.G. Chernoff, Indianapolis, IN.)

improvement in symptoms without additional recurrence for 14 months. Additionally, 2 patients with chronic temporomandibular joint syndrome had SVF injected directly and intravenously. One patient was symptom free at 1 year after injection. The second patient at 1 year reports ongoing pain, but reduced in intensity. Lander and colleagues showed improvement in patients with Peyronie's disease with SVF.[53] Interestingly, the pathophysiology of Peyronie's disease is similar to that of hypertrophic scarring and keloid formation.

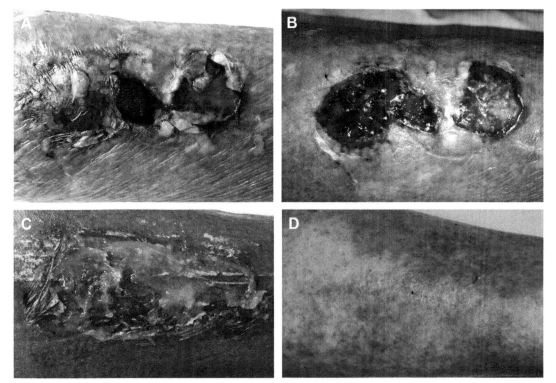

Fig. 6. Diabetic ulcer on the leg. (*A*) Study patient before treatment. (*B*) The same patients 4 weeks after intravenous infusion and local injection of stromal vascular fraction. (*C*) At 8 weeks after treatment. (*D*) At 16 weeks after treatment. (*Courtesy of* W.G. Chernoff, Indianapolis, IN.)

Stromal Vascular Fraction and the Treatment of Various Skin Conditions

The literature shows that scar formation may be prevented by inflammatory regulation.[54] The SVF was administered to a 6-month nonhealing diabetic leg ulcer (**Fig. 6**); interestingly, within 4 weeks, the periphery of the diabetic ulcer showed areas of epithelialization. By 16 weeks of injection and IV administration, the ulcer was totally reepithelialized. At the time of excising the recurring keloid, SVF was injected into the wound edges and given IV. **Fig. 7** shows the "4-time" previously excised recurring submental keloid. The patient is now 2 years after excision without recurrence. **Figs. 8** and **9** demonstrate

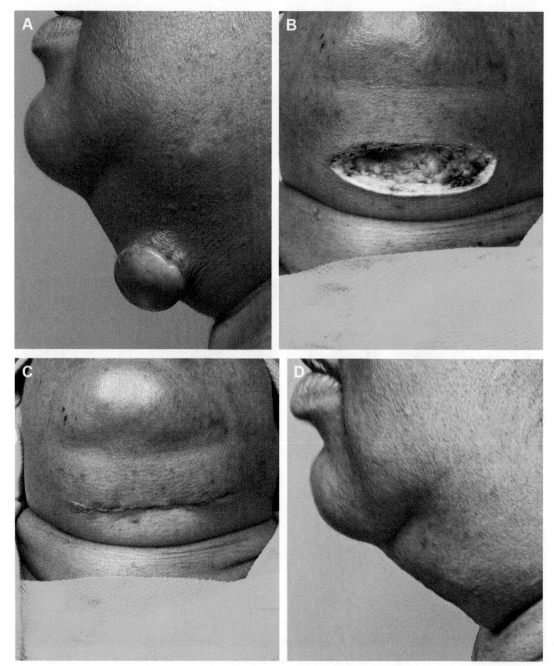

Fig. 7. Keloid scar. (*A*) Study patient before treatment, (*B*) Excision and deployment of stromal vascular fraction. (*C*) At 4 weeks after treatment. (*D*) At 2 years after treatment. (*Courtesy of* W.G. Chernoff, Indianapolis, IN.)

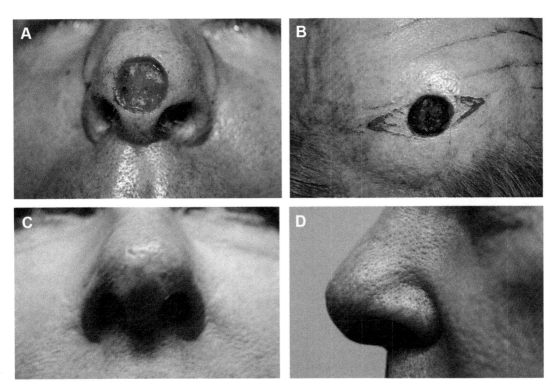

Fig. 8. Full- thickness skin graft. (*A*) Study patient before treatment. (*B*) Study patient before treatment. (*C*) At 1 year after intravenous infusion and local injection of stromal vascular fraction. (*D*) At 1 year after intravenous infusion and local injection of stromal vascular fraction. (*Courtesy of* W.G. Chernoff, Indianapolis, IN.)

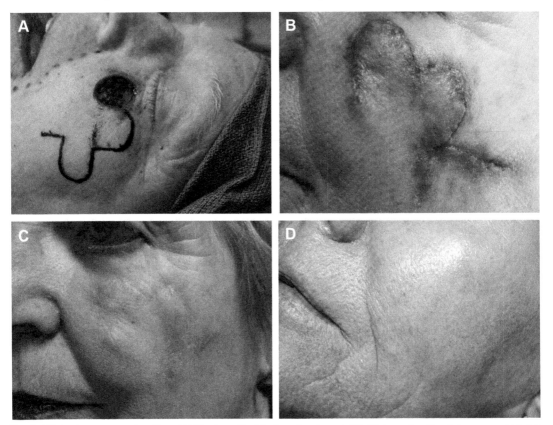

Fig. 9. Bilobed reconstruction flap. (*A*) Study patient before treatment. (*B*) At 4 weeks after intravenous infusion and local injection of stromal vascular fraction. (*C*) At 12 weeks after treatment. (*D*) At 1 year after treatment. (*Courtesy of* W.G. Chernoff, Indianapolis, IN.)

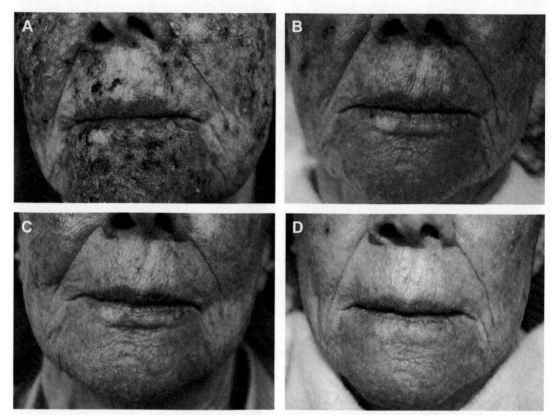

Fig. 10. Psoriasis. (*A*) Patient before treatment. (*B*) At 4 weeks after intravenous infusion and local injection of stromal vascular fraction. (*C*) At 12 weeks after treatment. (*D*) At 16 weeks after treatment. (*Courtesy of* W.G. Chernoff, Indianapolis, IN.)

results after a diabetic full-thickness nasal skin graft after basal cell carcinoma resection and a facial bilobe rotation flap patient after squamous cell carcinoma resection, respectively. There were no observed differences in healing with the full-thickness skin graft or the facial flap reconstructions. Although residual scars had an excellent cosmetic result, the patients did use other scar reduction therapies. Future double-blinded scar therapy studies using SVF are warranted. **Fig. 10** shows 2 patients with chronic psoriasis who had SVF injected locally and intravenously. At 4 months after injection and infusion of SVF, both patients reported clearing of symptoms. At 12 months status post deployment, both patients report ongoing reduced symptomatology.

CURRENT STROMAL VASCULAR FRACTION RESEARCH

SVF and mesenchymal stem cells have shown tremendous promise in regenerative therapy. The use of SVF in cosmetic and plastic surgery has

been well-documented. Yoshimura used SVF in conjunction with fat transfer to fortify the fat graft to improve uptake particularly in augmentation of breasts with fat, and coined the term cell-assisted lipotransfer.[55] A number of other CAL applications are under investigation, including therapy for facial, neck, hand, and buttock deployments. **Box 3** summarizes additional areas of research.

SUMMARY

The composition and safety of SVF, including mesenchymal stem cells, has been well-documented. Preliminary therapeutic studies have proven promising, and with further investigation and optimization of deployment, perhaps through regulation of NO production, SVF therapy will revolutionize the field of medicine. The fields of cellular therapy, regenerative medicine, and stem cell therapy continue to expand expanding, and although much work has been done, there is much work yet to be done.

<table>
<tr><td>

Box 3
Areas of current research

Wound healing
- Skin grafts
- Flap closures
- Diabetic ulcers
- Keloid scars
- Hypertrophic scars
- Burn wounds

Autoimmune conditions
- Hashimoto's thyroiditis
- Sjogren syndrome
- Keratoconjunctivitis sicca
- Psoriasis
- Rosacea
- Eczema

Inflammatory conditions
- Acne
- Temporomandibular joint syndrome
- Sinusitis

Degenerative
- Vaginal atrophy

Pain management
- Migraine headaches

Courtesy of W.G. Chernoff, Indianapolis, IN.

</td></tr>
</table>

REFERENCES

1. BermanM, Lander E, editors. The stem cell revolution. Bloomington (IN): Authorhouse; 2015.
2. Title 21 of the Code of Federal Regulations (CFR) Part 1271.
3. Pak J, Lee JH, Lee SH. Regenerative repair of damaged meniscus with autologous adipose-derived stem cells. Biomed Res Int 2014;2014:43602.
4. Cayci C, Carlsen BT. Osteoarthritis of the wrist. Plast Reconstr Surg 2014;13(3):605–15.
5. Chang H, Do BR, Che JH, et al. Safety of adipose-derive stem cells and collagenase in fat tissue preparation. Aesthetic Plast Surg 2013;37(4):802–8.
6. Pak J. Regeneration of human bones in hip osteonecrosis and human cartilage in knee osteoarthritis with autologous adipose-tissue derived stem cells: a case series. J Med Case Rep 2011;5:296.
7. Rodriguez JP, Murphy MP, Hong S, et al. Autologous stromal vascular fraction therapy for rheumatoid arthritis: rationale and clinical safety. Int Arch Med 2012;5:5.
8. Zellner J, Mueller M, Berner A, et al. Role of mesenchymal stem cells in tissue engineering of meniscus. J Biomed Mater Res A 2010;94(4):1150–61.
9. Koga H, Engebretsen L, Brinchman JE, et al. Mesenchymal stem cell based therapy for cartilage repair: a review. Knee Surg Sports Traumatol Arthrosc 2009;11:1289–97.
10. Centeno CJ, Busse D, Kisiday J, et al. Regeneration of meniscus cartilage in a knee treated with percutaneously implanted autologous mesenchymal cells. Med Hypotheses 2008;71(6):900–8.
11. Song M, Lim J, Yu HY, et al. Mesenchymal stem cell therapy alleviates interstitial cystitis by activating Wnt signaling pathway. Stem Cells Dev 2015;24(14):1648–57.
12. Riordan NH, Ichim TE, Min WP, et al. Non-expanded adipose stromal vascular fraction cell therapy for multiple sclerosis. J Transl Med 2009;7:29.
13. Zuk PA, Zhu M, Mizuno H, et al. Multi-lineage cells from human adipose tissue: implications for cell-based therapies. Tissue Eng 2001;7(2):211–28.
14. Harman R, Cowles B, Orava C, et al. A retrospective review of 60 case of joint injury in sport horses treated with adipose-derived stem and regenerative cell therapy. Vet Stem Intern Data 2006.
15. Melief SM, Zwaginga JJ, Fibbe WE, et al. Adipose tissue-derived multipotent stromal cells have a higher immunomodulatory capacity than their bone marrow-derived counterparts. Stem Cells Transl Med 2013;6:455–63.
16. Guo J, Nguyen A, Banyard DA, et al. Stromal vascular fraction: a regenerative reality? part 2: mechanisms of regenerative action. J Plast Reconstr Aesthet Surg 2016;69(2):180–8.
17. Nguyen A, Guo J, Banyard DA, et al. Stromal vascular fraction: a regenerative reality? Part 1: current concepts and review of the literature. J Plast Reconstr Aesthet Surg 2016;69(2):170–9.
18. Berman M, Lander E. A prospective study of autologous adipose-derived stromal vascular fraction using a special surgical processing system. AM J Cosm Surg 2017.
19. Human tissue intended for transplantation, 62 Fed. Reg. 40,429. July 29, 1997.
20. Arnold WP, Mittal CK, Katsuki S, et al. Nitric oxide activates guanylate cyclase and increases guanosine 3':5'-cyclic monophosphate levels in various tissue preparations. Proc Natl Acad Sci U S A 1977;74(8):3203–7.
21. Gaston B, Singel D, Doctor A, et al. S-nitrosothiol signaling in respiratory biology. Am J Respir Crit Care Med 2006;173(11):1186–93.

22. Lane P, Hao G, Gross SS. S-nitrosylation is emerging as a specific and fundamental post-translational protein modification: head-to-head comparison with O-phosphorylation. Sci STKE 2001;2001(86):RE1.

23. Bryan NS, Bian K, Murad F. Discovery of the nitric oxide signaling pathway and targets for drug development. Front Biosci 2009;14:1–18.

24. Porst H, Padma-Nathan H, Giuliano F, et al. Efficacy of tadalafil for the treatment of erectile dysfunction at 24 and 36 hours after dosing: a randomized controlled trial. Urology 2003;62(1):121–5 [discussion: 125–6].

25. Becker BF, Kupatt C, Massoudy P, et al. Reactive oxygen species and nitric oxide in myocardial ischemia and reperfusion. Z Kardiol 2000;89(Suppl 9):IX/88–91.

26. Hyde ER, Andrade F, Vaksman Z, et al. Metagenomic analysis of nitrate-reducing bacteria in the oral cavity: implications for nitric oxide homeostasis. PLoS One 2014;9(3):e88645.

27. Bryan NS, Tribble G, Angelov N. Oral microbiome and nitric oxide: the missing link in the management of blood pressure. Curr Hypertens Rep 2017;19(4):33.

28. Duncan C, Dougall H, Johnston P, et al. Chemical generation of nitric oxide in the mouth from the enterosalivary circulation of dietary nitrate. Nat Med 1995; 1(6):546–51.

29. Aicher A, Heeschen C, Mildner-Rihm C, et al. Essential role of endothelial nitric oxide synthase for mobilization of stem and progenitor cells. Nat Med 2003; 9(11):1370–6.

30. Mujoo K, Sharin VG, Bryan NS, et al. Role of nitric oxide signaling components in differentiation of embryonic stem cells into myocardial cells. Proc Natl Acad Sci U S A 2008;105(48):18924–9.

31. Thom SR, Bhopale VM, Velazquez OC, et al. Stem cell mobilization by hyperbaric oxygen. Am J Physiol Heart Circ Physiol 2006;290(4):H1378–86.

32. Egashira K, Inou T, Hirooka Y, et al. Effects of age on endothelium-dependent vasodilation of resistance coronary artery by acetylcholine in humans. Circulation 1993;88(1):77–81.

33. Taddei S, Virdis A, Ghiadoni L, et al. Age-related reduction of NO availability and oxidative stress in humans. Hypertension 2001;38(2):274–9.

34. Gerhard M, Roddy MA, Creager SJ, et al. Aging progressively impairs endothelium-dependent vasodilation in forearm resistance vessels of humans. Hypertension 1996;27(4):849–53.

35. Esper RJ, Nordaby RA, Vilariño JO, et al. Endothelial dysfunction: a comprehensive appraisal. Cardiovasc Diabetol 2006;5:4.

36. Ignarro LJ. Nitric oxide as a unique signaling molecule in the vascular system: a historical overview. J Physiol Pharmacol 2002;53(4 Pt 1):503–14.

37. Herman AG, Moncada S. Therapeutic potential of nitric oxide donors in the prevention and treatment of atherosclerosis. Eur Heart J 2005; 26(19):1945–55.

38. Ignarro LJ, Buga GM, Wood KS, et al. Endothelium-derived relaxing factor produced and released from artery and vein is nitric oxide. Proc Natl Acad Sci U S A 1987;84(24):9265–9.

39. Ma XL, Weyrich AS, Lefer DJ, et al. Diminished basal nitric oxide release after myocardial ischemia and reperfusion promotes neutrophil adherence to coronary endothelium. Circ Res 1993;72(2): 403–12.

40. Li J, Bombeck CA, Yang S, et al. Nitric oxide suppresses apoptosis via interrupting caspase activation and mitochondrial dysfunction in cultured hepatocytes. J Biol Chem 1999; 274(24):17325–33.

41. Zand J, Lanza F, Garg HK, et al. All-natural nitrite and nitrate containing dietary supplement promotes nitric oxide production and reduces triglycerides in humans. Nutr Res 2011;31(4):262–9.

42. Nagamani SC, Campeau PM, Shchelochkov OA, et al. Nitric-oxide supplementation for treatment of long-term complications in argininosuccinic aciduria. Am J Hum Genet 2012;90(5):836–46.

43. Houston M, Hays L. Acute effects of an oral nitric oxide supplement on blood pressure, endothelial function, and vascular compliance in hypertensive patients. J Clin Hypertens (Greenwich) 2014; 1716(7):524–9.

44. Biswas OS, Gonzalez VR, Schwarz ER. Effects of an oral nitric oxide supplement on functional capacity and blood pressure in adults with prehypertension. J Cardiovasc Pharmacol Ther 2014;20(1): 52–8.

45. Lee J, Kim HT, Solares GJ, et al. Caffeinated nitric oxide-releasing lozenge improves cycling time trial performance. Int J Sports Med 2015; 36(2):107–12.

46. Kurokawa I, Danby F, Danby FW, et al. New developments in our understanding of acne pathogenesis and treatment. Exp Dermatol 2009;18: 821–32.

47. Qin M, Pirouz A, Kim MH, et al. P acnes induces IL-1beta secretion via the NLRP3 inflammasome in human monocytes. J Invest Dermatol 2014;134(2): 381–8.

48. Bowe W, Kober M. Therapeutic update: acne. J Invest Dermatol 2014;13:235–8.

49. Jeremy AH, Holland DB, Roberts SG, et al. Inflammatory events are involved in acne lesion initiation. J Invest Dermatol 2003;121:20–7.

50. Kistowska M, Gehrke S, Jankovic D, et al. IL-beta drives inflammatory responses to P acnes in vitro and in vivo. J Invest Dermatol 2014;134: 677–85.

51. Contassot E. New insights into acne pathogenesis: P acnes activates the inflammasome. J Invest Dermatol 2014;134:677–85.

52. Lander EB, Berman MH, See JR. Stromal vascular fraction combined with shock wave for the treatment of Peyronie's disease. Plast Reconstr Surg Glob Open 2016;4(3):e631.

53. Liu S, Jiang L, Li H, et al. Mesenchymal stem cells prevent hypertrophic scar formation via inflammatory regulation when undergoing apoptosis. J Invest Dermatol 2014;134:2648–57.

54. Lee E. Effects of nitric oxide on carotid intima media thickness: a pilot study. Altern Ther Health Med 2016;22(S2):32–4.

55. Yoshimura K, Sato K, Aoi N, et al. Cell-assisted lipotransfer for cosmetic breast augmentation: supportive use of adipose-derived stem/stromal cells. Aesthetic Plast Surg 2008;32(1):48–55.

Mesenchymal Stem Cells and Stromal Vascular Fraction for Hair Loss
Current Status

Gorana Kuka Epstein, MD[a,b,c,*], Jeffrey S. Epstein, MD[d,e,f]

KEYWORDS

- Adipose-derived stem cells • Hair loss • Androgenic alopecia • Stromal vascular fraction
- Regenerative cell therapy

KEY POINTS

- Regenerative therapy has an expanding role in the treatment of various forms of alopecia.
- A review of the literature confirms the beneficial results of various cell therapies for such conditions as male and female androgenic alopecia and scarring alopecia.
- Adipose tissue allows for safe and easy access to regenerative cells and stromal vascular fraction and appears to be a low-risk harvesting procedure.
- The authors' experience shows positive indications for using purified fat and hair transplantation in certain hair loss conditions.

INTRODUCTION

Mesenchymal stromal cells (MSCs) are undifferentiated cells that are able to renew their population and become differentiated to produce all specialized cell types of the tissue from which they originate.[1,2] Apart from traditionally being isolated from the bone marrow, the first tissue from which stem cells were identified, MSCs have also been found in many other tissues, such as liver, cord blood, placenta, dental pulp, and adipose tissue.[2] Adipose-derived stromal cells (ADSCs) are easier to isolate and provide a higher number of stromal cells than bone marrow tissue.[3]

The main roles of MSCs are to maintain the stem cell niche, facilitate recovery after injury, and ensure homeostasis of organs and tissues.[4] ADSCs can differentiate into mesenchymal lineage cells but also secrete various cytokines and growth factors that have paracrine effects on surrounding cells: vascular endothelial growth factor (VEGF), hepatocyte growth factor (HGF), insulin-like growth factor (IGF), platelet-derived growth factors (PDGF), and others.[5,6] These factors seem to play a role in neovascularization, which is important in a variety of hair loss conditions.

Androgenic alopecia (AGA) remains the main cause of hair loss in both men and women.[7,8] The 2 medicines currently approved by the Food and Drug Administration for the treatment of AGA are finasteride (for men only) and minoxidil. Both carry untoward side effects and lack consistent efficacy.[9,10]

Disclosure: The authors have nothing to disclose.
[a] BelPrime Clinic, Department for Hair Restoration "Hair Center Serbia", Brane Crncevica 16, 11000 Belgrade, Serbia; [b] Department of Research, Foundation for Hair Restoration, 6280 Sunset Drive, Suite 504, Miami, FL 33143, USA; [c] Department of Research, Foundation for Hair Restoration, 60e 56th Street, New York, NY 10021, USA; [d] Foundation for Hair Restoration, 6280 Sunset Drive, Miami, FL 33143, USA; [e] Foundation for Hair Restoration, 6280 Sunset Drive, Suite 504, Miami, FL 33143, USA; [f] Foundation for Hair Restoration, 60e 56th Street, New York, NY 10021, USA
* Corresponding author. 6280 Sunset Drive, Suite 504, Miami, FL 33143.
E-mail address: gorana.kuka@me.com

Facial Plast Surg Clin N Am 26 (2018) 503–511
https://doi.org/10.1016/j.fsc.2018.06.010
1064-7406/18/Published by Elsevier Inc.

THE AUTHORS' RATIONALE

In the authors' earliest work with adipose tissue, they saw its distinct potential as an adjunct in hair transplantation surgery in the reconstruction of scalp scars. The growth of hair follicles transplanted into scars is usually lower than in normal scalp because of a thick collagen pattern and compromised blood supply in scar tissue. The authors' method is to pretreat scalp scars with autologous adipose tissue injections and then perform the hair transplant procedure 3 months later. Early on in their work, the authors were encouraged by the finding that during the creation of recipient sites into which the hair grafts would be inserted, the scar tissue would usually bleed more than untreated scar tissue, a benefit of the angiogenesis that took place due to the addition of adipose tissue. This pretransplant fat transfer technique was applied successfully in treating scars of a variety of causes: burns, chemical injury, surgical injury, physical trauma, and congenital scar conditions **(Fig. 1)**.

Based on the authors' observed benefits in these scar tissue cases, they decided to apply fat grafting for the treatment of AGA. Theoretically, adipose tissue could have the following beneficial effects.

Anti-inflammatory Effect

Many scarring and nonscarring types of alopecia have some degree of underlying inflammation. Mild perifollicular fibrosis and infiltrates have also been found in patients with androgenetic alopecia.[11] ADSCs may prevent further inflammation and possible damage to hair follicles through the enhancement of antioxidative and anti-inflammatory mechanisms. Their anti-inflammatory and immunomodulatory properties are reflected in their potential to inhibit maturation and production of cytokines and to impair the cytotoxic potential of natural killer cells and T lymphocytes.[12] Furthermore, ADSCs are able to inhibit the proliferation of B cells and their capacity to produce antibodies.[12]

Antiandrogen Effect

Areas affected with hair loss have higher levels of dihydrotestosterone (DHT), an androgen that causes hair loss. Finasteride decreases levels of DHT but also has potential side effects. The antiandrogen effect of adipose tissue derives from the

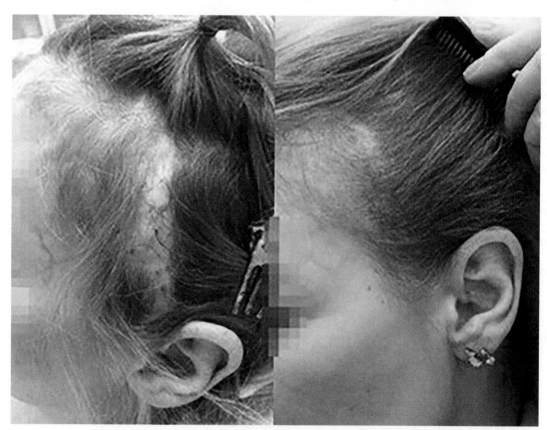

Fig. 1. A patient whose chemical injury in the temporal areas was pretreated with fat injections and then 3 months later underwent a hair transplant procedure.

isoenzyme aldo-keto reductase 1C2 (AKR1C2), which inactivates androgens by converting potent DHT into weak 3-alpha diol through 3-alpha reductase activity.[13] When injected into an area affected by hair loss, adipose tissue could exert an antiandrogen effect without systemic effects.

Re-creating Thickness of the Scalp

Hori and colleagues[14] published a paper 50 years ago that examined the variation in thickness of balding versus nonbalding scalp. It was observed that the thickness of the subdermis remains the same in early stages of male pattern baldness (MPB) and decreases sharply in advanced stages. This thinning of the adipose layer is a landmark of aging scalp, because it was even more notable in cadavers. By the injection of additional fat into the balding areas, a fuller subdermal layer of fat can be created, critical for the optimal growth of hair follicles, as well as to prevent its complete loss. Adipocytes act as a niche for hair follicles, increasing the skin's thickness and advancing the intradermal adipocyte layer during the anagen phase of hair growth that may counteract the hypothesis that the telogen phase may be due to an absence of adipose tissue, with the literature indicating that hair and adipose loss occur together. In addition, ADSCs and adipocytes regulate the hair cycle via the release of signaling molecules, that is, WNTs, platelet derived growth factors (PDGF), bone morphogenic proteins (BMPs), and fibroblast growth factors (FGFs).[15]

Mesenchymal Stem Cells

The paracrine characteristics of ADSCs may include the specific factors released by them, including VEGF, HGF, IGF, and PDGF, that have possible effects on hair regeneration.[16] There have been attempts to augment adipose retention and increase its survival on injection, limiting the need for repeat procedures. Zhu and colleagues[17] in an animal model showed improved retention of adipose tissue injected with cells versus adipose tissue alone at 6 and 9 months. Therefore, enriching adipose tissue with ADSCs could extend the benefits in treating hair loss.

Neovascularization

One myth about hair loss is that it is caused by poor blood circulation in the scalp. Although no scientific studies have been done, this poor circulation may in fact not be a myth but an important factor due to the decrease in the supply of blood that provides oxygen and nutrients to hair follicles. Several studies have shown that adipocytes can induce angiogenesis. Yuan and colleagues[18] presented that ADSCs may induce new blood vessel growth around and into the fat graft by releasing significant amounts of angiogenic growth factors, such as VEGF, HGF, basic fibroblast growth factor (BFGF). Magalon and colleagues,[19] in a study treating scleroderma patients with adipose-derived stromal vascular fraction (ADSVF) injections, noted that ADSVF may improve vasomotor tone and microvascular perfusion, which is consistent with one of the main properties of ADSVF, the promotion of vascular repair and angiogenesis.[4,20]

REVIEW OF THE LITERATURE

Although many studies have been published on hair regeneration using ADSCs in either cultured hair follicles or animal models, there have been only a few published on their application in human subjects. The authors searched PubMed up to November 2017 using terms related to hair regeneration: MSCs, ADSCs or ADSC-CM, alopecia, hair loss, restricted to human studies. Fukuoka and colleagues[21] were the first to use adipose-derived stem cell–conditioned medium (ADSC-CM) (AAPE; Prostemics, Seoul, Korea) in 22 patients (11 men and 11 women) injected intradermally every 3 to 5 weeks for 6 sessions. The ADSC-CM was delivered with a 31-gauge needle to provide 0.02 mL/cm^2 of solution with a total of 3 to 4 mL injected. Finasteride was administered to 6 of the 11 male patients. Trichograms were taken before and then 7 to 12 months after the initial treatment. Ten of the 22 patients had a half-side comparison study, receiving ADSC-CM treatment on the left side and placebo (saline injection) treatment on the right. The mean increase in number of hairs was 29 ± 4.1 in men and 15.6 ± 4.2 in women, with no significant difference observed between the finasteride and nonfinasteride group. In the half-side comparison study, the number of hairs was significantly higher in the treated versus placebo side.

In 2017, Fukuoka and colleagues[22] conducted another study with the same medium in 21 patients (16 men and 5 women) whereby injections were done in the same manner. After 3 months, there was a reported increase in the number of hairs from baseline of 141.2 ± 31.4 in men and 109.8 ± 43.5 in women. Also reported was that patients were often able to notice changes in hair quality and in reduction in area of the extent of thinning hair through photographs after 4 to 5 treatments. Similar to the prior study, 10 patients had a half-side comparison study, whereby saline was injected as a placebo. There was a significant difference in increased hair counts between the treatment and placebo sides (18.4 ± 9.4 vs 6.5 ± 11.7).

Shin and colleagues[23] published a retrospective case study on the clinical use of the same media of adipose tissue–derived stem cells in female pattern hair loss by analysis of patient medical records and phototrichographic images. This retrospective observational study of outcomes in 27 patients with female pattern hair loss treated with ADSC-CM showed efficacy after 12 weeks of therapy. Hair density increased from 105.4 to 122.7 hairs per squared centimeter, whereas hair thickness increased from 57.5 to 64.0 μm.

Shin and colleagues[11] assessed the effect of ADSC-CM in AGA in a study of 27 women and 25 men. Patients received ADSC-CM by microneedle roller or mesotherapy gun weekly for 12 weeks and were followed for 1 year. After 12 weeks of therapy, hair density increased from 105.4 to 122.7 counts per squared centimeter, whereas mean hair thickness increased from 57.5 to 64.0 μm. In men specifically, this hair density increased from 97.7 to 108.1 counts per squared centimeter, and mean hair thickness increased from 65.4 to 71.8 μm. These effects were maintained for the full year, and no severe adverse reactions were reported. This study had a split-scalp study subgroup on 6 patients with MPB, using ADSC-CM on the test side and the same medium without ADSCs as a control. After 12 weeks of therapy, the total hair count in a circle 1 cm in diameter was significantly higher on the treated side ($P = .0010$); however, the mean hair diameter did not significantly differ between the sides.

Apart from ADSC-CM application, there was one study whereby stromal vascular fraction (SVF) with autologous adipose tissue was done in 9 patients (8 men and 1 woman).[24] The SVF was obtained from lipoaspirate processed by the Kerastem Celution System (Kerastem LLS, Solana Beach, CA, USA), whereas adipose tissue was purified by the Puregraft system (Puregraft LLC, Solana Beach, CA, USA) and injected separately. The mixture of adipose tissue, SVF, and lactated Ringer solution was injected in a fanlike pattern in the subcutaneous layer of the scalp using a 1.0-mL Luer Lock syringe attached to a 1.2-mm cannula to apply 1.0 mL of the mixture per square centimeter of scalp. One patient was treated with adipose injections only, whereas a split-scalp procedure was done using saline injection as a control. All male patients were in the Norwood 3 stage of hair loss, whereas no staging was available for the female patient. Follow-up was done by global photography, and macrophotography was done using the FotofinderMediscope Selective System, with results analyzed by Fotofinder System TrichoScale software (Fotofinder,

Columbia, MD, USA). Six-month follow-up data were available for 6 patients. In patients who received fat plus SVF, a mean increase of 31 hairs per squared centimeter (23% relative percentage increase) was documented, whereas in the one subject who received fat alone a mean increase of 14 hairs per squared centimeter of scalp was noted. In one split-scalp patient, the treatment area had an increase of 44.1 hairs per squared centimeter of scalp compared with the area receiving placebo that had a mean increase of 1.33 hairs per squared centimeter. Despite some limitations of the study (small sample size, poor follow-up data, nonblinded analysis), this initial study shows that SVF with fat injection is a safe and promising alternative approach to treating hair loss in men and women.

Apart from treating AGA, Dini and colleagues[25] presented a case of a female patient with alopecia areata of the left eyebrow treated with autologous fat transplantation. A marked improvement was noted in the atrophic scar, while hair regrowth was observed at 3 months (Fig. 2). Cho and colleagues[26] described a case of a woman suffering from scleroderma-induced atrophic alopecia who presented with a 3 × 4-cm alopecic patch on the frontal scalp. Two fat injections were performed 3 months apart, and hair growth was noticed 3 months after the second treatment.

Gentile and colleagues[27] published a study on treating 23 patients with andogenetic alopecia Norwood 3 to 5 with isolated stem cells from human follicles (HFSCs). Cells were isolated with a device called the Rigenaracons (CE certified class I; HBW srl, Turin, Italy) that disaggregates a strip of scalp from the back of the head (the usual "donor" area for a hair transplant, an area where hair follicles are not affected by DHT) under sterile conditions in 1.2 cc of physiologic solution. After 60 seconds of centrifugation at 80 rpm, a cell suspension was obtained and injected into the scalp by an Ultim gun (Anti-Aging Medical Systems, Montrodat, France) in 2 sessions spaced 60 days apart. Apart from the treatment area, another zone served as a control (saline injections). Follow-up was done by global, but not standardized, photography. Twenty-three weeks after the treatment, a 29% ± 5% increase in hair density was noted compared with a less than 1% increase noted in the placebo area. It is unclear how the increase in hair count was determined because no macrophotography was done. However, on global photographs, an improvement can be noted. This study is the first with HFSCs that showed a positive therapeutic effect on male AGA.

Zanzottera and colleagues[28] conducted a pilot study to assess the application of the same cellular

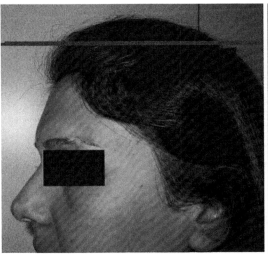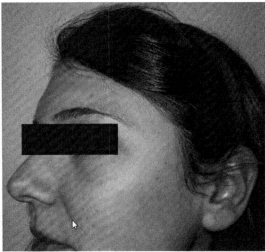

Fig. 2. A patient with alopecic eyebrow before and 3 months after adipose tissue injections. (*From* Dini M, Mori A. Eyebrow regrowth in patient with atrophic scarring alopecia treated with an autologous fat graft. Derm Surg 2014;40(8);926–8; with permission.)

suspension in its impact on wound healing and survival of transplanted hairs after a hair transplant procedure. At the conclusion of the hair transplant procedure, the adipose tissue recovered from the discarded donor material during graft preparation was processed using the Rigenera system (Human Brain Wave srl, Torino, Italy). This cell suspension was then injected subcutaneously and spread out over the recipient sites before and after the graft insertion. Three subjects were monitored after 5 days, 2 weeks, and 1 month. Two weeks after the procedure, healing of the microwounds was complete, and the hair continued growing, atypical after most hair transplant procedures, where the transplanted hairs typically fall out before starting to regrow 3 to 4 months later. The investigators also reported a low level of pain and edema in these patients. This study is a very small study, and more complete clinical work is necessary to better determine if and how this cell suspension improves hair transplantation results.

CURRENT STUDIES

A search of the terms "stem cells" and "hair loss" on www.clinicaltrials.gov resulted in reporting 6 studies using SVF to treat either AGA or alopecia areata (**Table 1**).

The only study completed to date is STYLE-Transplantation of Cell Enriched Adipose Tissue For Follicular Niche Stimulation in Early Androgenetic Alopecia. This trial was a randomized, blinded, controlled, multicentered trial wherein 71 subjects, men and women, were randomized into 4 groups: Puregraft fat enriched with high dose

of adipose-derived regenerative cells (ADRCs, $1.0 \times 10^6/cm^2$), Puregraft fat enriched with low dose of ADRCs ($0.5 \times 10^6/cm^2$), Puregraft fat alone, and saline injections only, in the ratio of 2:2:2:1. ADRCs were obtained by Kerastem Celution device (Kerastem LLS), from the patient's own adipose tissue, while fat was purified by the Puregraft system (Puregraft LLC). The fat was delivered into the subdermal layer by cannula ($0.1 \ mL/cm^2$), and the cells were delivered by 22-gauge needle injections ($0.1 \ mL/cm^2$) into a 40-cm² sized area. Follow-up was done by global and macrophotography at weeks 6, 12, 24, and 52. Although data through week 52 are still pending, the 24-week results were presented by the first author of this article at the International Society of Hair Restoration Surgery Annual Meeting in Prague in October 2017.[29,30] At 24 weeks, there was an absolute mean change in terminal hairs from baseline of 29 hairs per squared centimeter, compared with control (a 16% point delta) in men with Norwood Class 3 hair loss who received Puregraft fat enriched with low-dose ADRCs. No serious adverse events occurred.

AUTHORS' EXPERIENCE

Although the regulation on the use of SVF in the United States is still pending, the authors of this article began applying adipose injections for various types of alopecias. The authors are treating both men and women with either adipose tissue injections alone or with a 4:1 mixture of adipose tissue to platelet-rich plasma (PRP). To date, this therapy has been applied to conditions

Table 1
Current studies listed on www.clinicaltrials.gov on the use of stromal vascular fraction to treat androgenic alopecia or alopecia areata

Study Title and Trial Number	Conditions	Interventions	Outcome Measures	Number Enrolled	Locations
Stem Cell Educator Therapy in Alopecia Areata NCT01673789	Alopecia areata	Device: stem cell educator	Feasibility and efficacy of stem cell educator therapy in alopecia areata	30	The First Hospital of Hebei Medical University Shijiazhuang, Hebei, China
The Effect of Allogeneic Human Adipose-Derived Stem Cell Component on Androgenic Alopecia NCT02594046	AGA	Other: stem cell component extract	Change of total hair counts by phototrichogram	38	
Adipose Tissue-Derived Stem Cell-Based Hair Restoration therapy for Androgenetic Alopecia NCT02865421	Hair restoration using autologous mesenchymal stem cells	Drug: stem cells Drug: PRP	Pull test Trichoscan	88	
Biocellular-Cellular Regenerative Treatment Scarring Alopecia and Alopecia Areata NCT03078686	Alopecia areata Scarring areata	Procedure: tSVF by lipoaspiration Procedure: PRP concentration Procedure: emulsification tSVF	Safety of intervention hair growth assessment Photographic assessment scalp hair	60	• Kenneth Williams, DO Irvine, CA, USA • Regeneris, Medical North Attleboro, MA, USA • Regenevita LLC Stevensville, MT, USA
Point-of-Care Adipose-Derived Cells for Hair Growth NCT02729415	Androgenetic alopecia	Procedure: SVF cells Procedure liposuction Other: hair measurements	• Incidence of treatment-emergent adverse events • Growth of new hair from baseline to 6 wk, 3 mo, and 6 mo • Change in hair thickness from baseline to 6 wk, 3 mo, and 6 mo	8	• University of Florida, Gainesville, FL, USA
AGA Biocellular Stem/Stromal Hair Regenerative Study NCT02849470	Hair disease	• Procedure: intradermal injection in hair loss • Procedure: PRP • Procedure: adipose-derived stem/stromal cells	• Safety-tolerability assess of SAE/AE assessment of SAE/AES • Hair growth trichogram • Hair density trichogram	60	• Kenneth Williams, DO, Irvine, CA, USA

Abbreviations: AE, adverse event; AES, adverse events; SAE, serious adverse events; tSVF, tissue stromal vascular fraction.

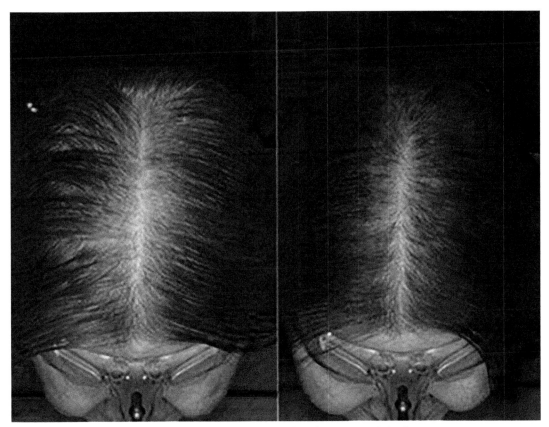

Fig. 3. A 57-year old female patient with hair loss treated by adipose tissue injections.

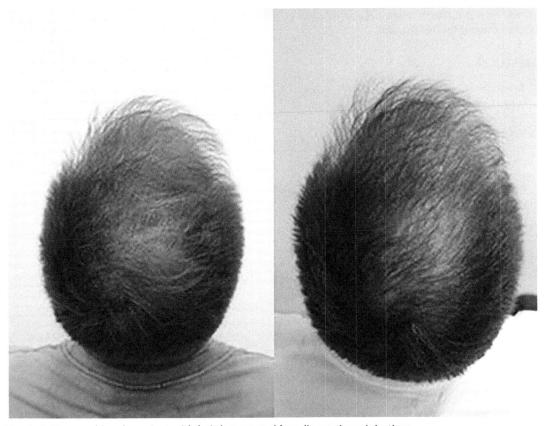

Fig. 4. A 28-year old male patient with hair loss treated by adipose tissue injections.

such as AGA, frontal fibrosing alopecia, lichen planopilaris, and alopecia totalis. The authors' method consists of harvesting fat with liposuction and processing it with the Puregraft system and then injecting it by cannula into the subcutaneous layer of the scalp. An amount of 0.1 to 0.2 cc of fat is injected per squared centimeter, and in certain conditions where scarring is encountered, there is a physical role of the cannula movements in breaking up the fibrous tissue, which is then further improved by the addition of the adipose tissue. Although still in the stage of collecting data, this therapy has proven to be safe, with improvements in overall appearance of the hair documented with photography (**Figs. 3** and **4**).

SUMMARY

Adipose tissue, as the easiest accessible source of mesenchymal stem cells, has emerged as a new therapeutic option for hair loss. The regenerating effects of ADSC-CM have been demonstrated by several clinical studies. Adipose-derived stem cells offer a huge potential for hair regeneration. It is up to future studies to establish more definitive protocols not only in the isolation of ADSCs but also in its application and answer dilemmas on their effectiveness. Based on initial work and the science behind it, the authors believe there is a definite potential for this therapy.

REFERENCES

1. Tabatabaei Qomi R, Sheykhhasan M. Adipose-derived stromal cell in regenerative medicine: a review. World J Stem Cells 2017;9(8):107–17.
2. Marquez-Curtis LA, Janowska-Wieczorek A, McGann LE, et al. Mesenchymal stromal cells derived from various tissues: biological, clinical and cryopreservation aspects. Cryobiology 2015; 71:181–97.
3. Sheykhhasan M, Qomi RT, Ghiasi M. Fibrin scaffolds designing in order to human adipose-derived mesenchymal stem cells differentiation to chondrocytes in the presence of TGF-β3. Int J Stem Cells 2015;8:219–27.
4. Rehman J, Traktuev D, Li J, et al. Secretion of angiogenic and antiapoptotic factors by human adipose stromal cells. Circulation 2004;109:1292–8.
5. Kinniard T, Stabile E, Burnett MS, et al. Narrow-derived stromal cells express gene encoding a broad spectrum of arteriogenic cytokines and promote in vitro and in vivo arteriogenesis through paracrine mechanisms. Circ Res 2004;94:678–85.
6. Whiting DA. Scalp biopsy as a diagnostic and prognostic tool in androgenetic alopecia. Dermatol Ther 1998;8:24–33.
7. Otberg N, Finner AM, Shapiro J. Androgenetic alopecia. Endocrinol Metab Clin North Am 2007;36(2): 379–98.
8. Dinh QQ, Sinclair R. Female pattern hair loss: current treatment concepts. Clin Interv Aging 2007; 2(2):189–99.
9. Ross EK, Shapiro J. Management of hair loss. Dermatol Clin 2005;23(2):227–43.
10. Mysore V. Finasteride and sexual side effects. Indian Dermatol Online J 2012;23(2):227–43.
11. Shin H, Won CH, Chung WK, et al. Up-to-date clinical trials of hair regeneration using conditioned media of adipose-derived stem cells in male and female pattern hair loss. Curr Stem Cell Res Ther 2017;12(7):524–30.
12. Zhao S, Wehner R, Bornhäuser M, et al. Immunomodulatory properties of mesenchymal stromal cells and their therapeutic consequences for immune-mediated disorders. Stem Cells Dev 2010;19(5): 607–14.
13. O'Reilly MW, House PJ, Tomlinson JW. Understanding androgen action in adipose tissue. J Steroid Biochem Mol Biol 2014;143:277–84.
14. Hori H, Moretti G, Rebora A, et al. The thickness of human scalp:normal and bald. J Invest Dermatol 1972;6:396–9.
15. Festa E, Fretz J, Berry R, et al. Adipocyte lineage cells contribute to the skin stem cell niche to drive hair cycling. Cell 2011;146(5):761–71.
16. Anderi R, Makdissy N, Rizk F, et al. Hair quality improvement in alopecia patients following adipose-derived stem cell treatment. JPRAS Open 2017.
17. Zhu M, Zhou Z, Chen Y, et al. Supplementation of fat grafts with adipose –derived regenerative cells improves long-term graft retention. Ann Plast Surg 2010;64:222–8.
18. Yuan Y, Gao J, Liu L, et al. Role of adipose-derived stem cells in enhancing angiogenesis early after aspirated fat transplantation: induction or differentiation? Cell Biol Int 2013;37(6):547–50.
19. Magalon G, Daumas A, Sautereau N, et al. Regenerative approach to scleroderma with fat grafting. Clin Plast Surg 2015;42:353–64.
20. Nakagami H, Maeda K, Morishita R, et al. Novel autologous cell therapy in ischemic limb disease through growth factor secretion by cultured adipose tissue-derived stromal cells. Arterioscler Thromb Vasc Biol 2005;25:2542–7.
21. Fukuoka H, Suga H. Hair regeneration treatment using adipose-derived stem cell conditioned medium: follow-up with trichograms. Eplasty 2015;15:e10.
22. Fukuoka H, Narita K, Suga H. Hair regeneration therapy using proteins secreted by adipose-derived stem cells. Curr Stem Cell Res Ther 2017; 12:531–4.
23. Shin H, Ryu HH, Kwon O, et al. Clinical use of conditioned media of adipose tissue-derived stem cells in

female pattern hair loss: a retrospective case series study. Int J Dermatol 2015;54(6):730–5.

24. Perez-Meza D, Ziering C, Sforza M, et al. Hair follicle growth by stromal vascular fraction-enhanced adipose transplantation in baldness. Stem Cells Cloning 2017;10:1–10.

25. Dini M, Mori A, Quattrini Li A. Eyebrow regrowth in patient with atrophic scarring alopecia treated with an autologous fat graft. Dermatol Surg 2014;40(8): 926–8.

26. Cho SB, Roh MR, Chung KY. Recovery of scleroderma-induced atrophic alopecia by autologous fat transplantation. Dermatol Surg 2010;36: 2061–3.

27. Gentile P, Scioli MG, Bielli A, et al. Stem cells from human hair follicles: first mechanical isolation for immediate autologous clinical use in androgenetic alopecia and hair loss. Stem Cell Investig 2017;4:58.

28. Zanzottera F, Lavezzari E, Trovato L, et al. Adipose derived stem cells and growth factors applied on hair transplantation follow-up of clinical outcome. J Chem Dermatol Sci Appl 2014;4:268–74.

29. Kuka Epstein G, Epstein J, Washenik K, et al. Transplantation of cell enriched adipose tissue for follicular niche stimulation in early androgenetic alopecia. Presented at annual meeting of the International Society of Hair Restoration Surgery ISHRS meeting, Prague, Check Republic, 2017.

30. Li Y, Yan B, Wang H, et al. Hair regrowth in alopecia areata patients following Stem Cell Educator therapy. BMC Med 2015;13:87.

Mesothelial Stem Cells and Stromal Vascular Fraction for Skin Rejuvenation

David A. Wolf, MD, EE[a,b,c], William Beeson, MD[d,e,f,*,1],
John D. Rachel, MD[g,2], Gregory S. Keller, MD[h,i,3],
C. William Hanke, MD, MPH[j,k,l,m,n], Jill Waibel, MD[o,p,q],
Matt Leavitt, DO[r,s,t,u], Michael Sacopulos, JD[v]

KEYWORDS

- Mesenchymal stem cells • Adipose-derived stem cells • Growth factors
- Stromal vascular fraction (SVF) • Regenerative medicine

KEY POINTS

- The process of extracting, concentrating, and administering stem cells has been shown in clinical trials to exhibit beneficial effects in many degenerative conditions.
- Cellular therapies have shown great promise for skin rejuvenation, hair restoration, and many other clinical applications in other areas of medicine.
- Growing evidence now suggests that the 2 aging processes have converging biochemical and molecular pathways that lead to photoaging of skin.
- The common mechanisms of the 2 aging processes may provide several unique opportunities to develop antiaging therapies.
- Although it is unclear how large proteins, such as growth factors, are able to penetrate the skin and become pharmacologically effective, early objective clinical studies and subjective observations indicate that these cosmeceutical products may potentially reduce signs of facial aging.

Disclosure: The authors have nothing to disclose.
[a] Johnson Space Center, Houston, TX, USA; [b] EarthTomorrow, Inc, 1714 Neptune Lane, Houston, TX 77062, USA; [c] Purdue University, West Lafayette, IN, USA; [d] Facial Plastics, Indianapolis, IN, USA; [e] Department of Dermatology, Indiana University School of Medicine, Indianapolis, IN, USA; [f] Department of Otolaryngology–Head and Neck Surgery, Indiana University School of Medicine, Indianapolis, IN, USA; [g] Facial Plastics, Chicago, IL, USA; [h] Facial Plastics, Santa Barbara, CA, USA; [i] Facial Plastics, Los Angeles, CA, USA; [j] Dermatology, Indianapolis, IN, USA; [k] Laser and Skin Center of Indiana, 13400 North Meridian Street, Suite 290, Carmel, IN 46032, USA; [l] ACGME Micrographic Surgery, Dermatologic Oncology Fellowship Training Program, St. Vincent Hospital, Indianapolis, IN, USA; [m] University of Iowa-Carver College of Medicine, Iowa City, IA, USA; [n] University of Cincinnati College of Medicine, Cincinnati, OH, USA; [o] Dermatology, Miami Dermatology and Laser Institute, 7800 Southwest 87th Avenue, Suite B200, Miami, FL 33173, USA; [p] Baptist Hospital of Miami, Miami, FL, USA; [q] Miller School of Medicine, University of Miami, Miami, FL, USA; [r] Dermatology, Orlando, FL, USA; [s] Advanced Dermatology and Cosmetic Surgery, The Hair Foundation, 260 Lookout Place Suite 103, Maitland, FL 32751, USA; [t] University of Central Florida, 6850 Lake Nona Boulevard, Orlando, FL 32827, USA; [u] Nova Southeastern University, 4850 Millenium Boulevard, Orlando, FL 32839, USA; [v] Medical Risk Management, Medical Risk Institute, 676 Ohio Street, Terre Haute, IN 47807, USA
[1] Present address: 3933 Kitty Hawk Court, Carmel, IN 46033.
[2] Present address: 2350 Ravine Way # 400 Glenview, IL 60025.
[3] Present address: 221 West Pueblo Street, Suite A, Santa Barbara, CA 93105.
* Corresponding author. 10500 Cross Point Boulevard, Indianapolis, IN 46256.
E-mail address: bill@beeson.com

Facial Plast Surg Clin N Am 26 (2018) 513–532
https://doi.org/10.1016/j.fsc.2018.06.011

INTRODUCTION

The use of stem cells in regenerative medicine and specifically in facial rejuvenation is thought provoking and controversial. Stem cells have a natural ability to repair damaged tissue. They are inherent in most tissues of the body and function in a restorative capacity in many tissues, such as the skin, where stem cells facilitate a rejuvenation of epidermal basal cell layers every day and in the intestinal tract, where mucosal lining tissues are replaced approximately every 4 days. In the case of degenerative diseases, these cells are not activated quickly enough to fully repair damaged tissue. The process of extracting, concentrating, and administering these stem cells has been shown in clinical trials to exhibit beneficial effects in many degenerative conditions. In addition, cellular therapies have shown great promise for skin rejuvenation, hair restoration, and many other clinical applications in other areas of medicine.

Surgeons have previously believed that damaged or diseased human tissue could be replaced only by donor transplants or, in select cases, alloplastic implants. Today there is increased emphasis on tissue engineering and regenerative medicine. Tissue engineering provides a more advanced approach in which organs or tissues can be repaired, replaced, or regenerated for a more focused treatment approach. Tissue engineering combines the principles of bioengineering, cell transplantation, biomaterial engineering, and surgery.

CATEGORIES OF STEM CELLS

Stem cells possess 2 important characteristics: they can renew themselves and they can give rise to specialized cell types. Essentially, there are 2 different classifications of stem cells: embryonic and adult. Embryonic stem cells (ESCs) are isolated from the inner cell mass of blastocysts. Adult stem cells have been identified in many organs and tissues and reside in a specific area of each tissue called a "stem cell niche." There are 3 different types of adult stem cells: pluripotent, multipotent, and unipotent. Pluripotent stem cells, such as embryonic or induced pluripotent stem cells (iPSCs), have the capacity to generate into tissue from any of the 3 germ layers. The risk for potential teratoma formation has impacted their clinical use. Multipotent stem cells, such as mesenchymal stromal cells, lack this negative effect and have the capacity to differentiate into a more limited number of closely related cells. Unipotent stem cells, although retaining the ability to self-renew, can produce only 1 cell type. This group plays a critical role in normal tissue homeostasis. The stem cells we are talking about for clinical therapies are essentially the multipotent type of stem cells that are derived from mesoderm.[1–3]

In the field of regenerative medicine, there is a need for a reliable source of stem cells in addition to biomaterial scaffolds and cytokine growth factors. Candidates include ESCs, iPSCs, and postnatal adult stem cells. ESCs and iPSCs have significant therapeutic potential, because of their auto reproducibility and their pluripotentiality. However, ethical considerations, cell regulations, and genetic manipulation limit their practical use. Postnatal adult stem cells are immunocompatible and are not fraught with ethical issues regarding their use. Postnatal adult stem cells can be obtained from bone marrow stroma, adipose tissue, dentition, skin, and a multitude of other tissues. They are termed mesenchymal stem cells (MSCs) and have adipogenic, osteogenic, chondrogenic, myogenic, and neurogenic potential.[2–5]

Induced Pluripotent Stem Cells

Ethical concerns associated with the use of ESCs spurred research efforts that would convert adult stem cells into pluripotent cells. In 2006, Shinya Yamanaka (Kyoto, Japan) altered the genes in specialized adult male cells to cause dedifferentiation and return to an embryonic–like stem cell state. The mouse somatic cells were reprogrammed to activate a combination of transcription factors. The cells were termed "induced pluripotent stem cells" (iPSCs). Yamanaka was awarded the Noble Prize "for the discovery that mature cells could be reprogrammed to become pluripotent." In 2007, both Yamanaka and James Thomas (University of Wisconsin) independently developed techniques to reprogram human cells into iPSCs.[6]

Typically, viruses are used to genomically alter the cell to produce iPSCs. There were concerns that this manipulation could trigger the expression of oncogenes (cancer-causing genes). However, in 2008, techniques were discovered that removed oncogenes after induction of pluripotency. This opened the door for the potential use of iPSCs in human disease.[7] Considerable research into anti-aging has focused on using iPSCs to reprogram cell senescence. However, it has been noted that altering of iPSCs at a cellular level also allows for the stimulation of collagen synthesis. This potential for iPSCs to generate collagen has significant implications in the field of aesthetic surgery (**Box 1**).

In the past, there was no standard nomenclature and no standard, accepted method for identifying stem cells. For this reason, in 2006, the

> **Box 1**
> **Stem cell overview**
>
> Stem cells have remarkable potential to develop into many different cell types.
>
> Stem cells have 2 important characteristics:
>
> 1. They can renew themselves
> 2. They can give rise to specialized cell types
>
> There are 2 types of stem cells:
>
> 1. Embryonic stem cells are isolated from the inner cell mass of blastocysts
> 2. Adult stem cells have been identified in many organs and tissues and reside in a specific area of each tissue called a "stem cell niche"
>
> The classic definition of a stem cell requires that it possess 5 properties:
>
> Self-renewal: ability to go through numerous cell divisions while maintaining the undifferentiated state
>
> Potency: capacity to differentiate into specialized cell types
>
> Pluripotent: ability to give rise to any mature cell type
>
> Multipotent: ability to develop into more than 1 cell type, but only those of a closely related family of cells
>
> Unipotent: ability to produce only 1 cell type but have property of self-renewal (multipotent and unipotent progenitor cells are often referred to as stem cells)

International Society for Cellular Therapy proposed a set of minimum criteria for identifying cells as stem cells.[8] These cells needed to adhere to plastic in culture and express certain surface molecules while lacking expression of others. In 2013, additional surface markers were added that should be expressed more than 80% of the time on the surface of stem cells, whereas certain negative markers should be expressed on fewer than 2% of the cells.[9,10] The viability of isolated cells needed to exceed 70% and have the presence of at least 2 positive and 2 negative markers for establishing a phenotype. In addition, the cells must possess the ability to differentiate into osteoblasts, adipocytes, and chondroblasts. The International Society for Cellular Therapy recommends calling these cells from any source "multipotent mesenchymal stromal cells."

Autologous (from the same organism) -derived mesenchymal stromal cells require initial harvesting of tissue, which is usually via an invasive procedure. In the case of adipose tissue, this is usually by means of a direct surgical resection of adipose tissue or through liposuction aspirate. In the case of bone marrow–derived tissue, this is by means of an invasive bone marrow biopsy. In addition, the tissue has to be processed, taking several hours in the case of stromal vascular fraction (SVF) and days to weeks in the case of culturing and expanding cells.

Allogeneic (from multiple organisms within the same species) -derived mesenchymal stromal cells raise immunomodulatory concerns, such as graft versus host disease. In addition, there are concerns over communicable disease being transferred from donors to recipient.

In the case of adult stem cells, whether they are derived as autologous tissue from an individual patient or allogenically derived tissue from multiple donors, there is the concern of decreasing "stemness" of the cells. Many feel that over time, the potency or the "stemness" of the cells decreases, such that cells derived from older patients are less robust and therefore less clinically effective than cells derived from younger individuals.[11,12]

Pluripotent stem cells have significant therapeutic potential, because of their ability to differentiate into virtually any cell type. Pluripotent stem cells are isolated in 3 ways[1]: directly from human embryos (ESCs),[2] from cloned embryos through somatic cell nuclear transfer, or[3] from adult cells reprogrammed to a pluripotent state, usually by means of a virus inserted into the cell DNA resulting in genetic "reprograming" of the cell (iPSCs). Pluripotent stem cell work can involve the creation and destruction of embryos, and concerns have been raised regarding the potential for uncontrolled growth (such as teratomas). Their use has been complicated by not only significant technical challenges, but also because of serious ethical concerns.[1,13,14]

SOURCES OF STEM CELLS

Stem cells obtained from adult adipose tissue (adipose-derived stem cells or "ASCs" or "ADSCs," as they are commonly designated) are one of the most popular adult stem cell populations currently being used in stem cell research. This novel adult stem cell population isolated from adipose tissue was first described by researchers at the University of California Los Angeles in 2002. Their multilineage mesodermal, ectodermal, and endodermal potential conceivably make the ASC an alternate to pluripotent ESCs in clinical applications.[15] There are only 2 categories of stem cells: the ESC and the postnatal stem cell (ie, adult stem cell). The embryonic stem cell is derived from the embryo's blastocyst inner cell mass.

The adult stem cell is derived from postnatal tissues and can include fetal-derived stem cells and umbilical cord blood stem cells.[1–3]

Mizuno and others[14] have shown that cells obtained from human liposuction fat aspirates can also differentiate into adipogenic, osteogenic, chondrogenic, and myogenic cells in a lineage-specific culture medium. Such cells are termed ASCs.[14,16] Multiple studies have shown that there is no difference in MSCs obtained from bone marrow or adipose tissue with regard to fibroblast-like morphology, immune phenotype, colony frequency, and differentiation capacity.[17]

There are several reasons to suggest ASCs for regenerative-based soft tissue therapies. First is their multipotentiality, especially their proclivity for adipose differentiation. It is relatively simple to achieve a high level of adipose differentiation of ASCs in vitro, and many studies have developed methods to use them in vivo. Second, ASCs appear to potentiate angiogenesis and vasculogenesis. Third, surgeons have a significant familiarity and comfort level with the harvest and manipulation of adipose tissue.

STRUCTURE AND CELLULAR COMPOSITION OF SKIN AS IT RELATES TO DERMATOLOGIC AGING AND REGENERATIVE MEDICINE

MSCs derived from adipose tissue provide signaling to tissues that serves to adjust immune response, cell differentiation, migration, and enzymatic reactions. ASCs play a significant role in the maintenance of dermal and epidermal homeostasis.[11] To better understand this phenomenon, it is important to have a knowledge of dermatologic aging as well as skin structure and cellular composition as it relates to regenerative medicine.

Dermatologic aging is a result of deficiencies in intrinsic cellular processes (DNA repair and instability, mitochondrial function, control over cellular metabolism, and control over cell cycle and apoptosis) and changes in epidermal homeostasis (integrity of extracellular matrix). These physiologic changes in the skin are exemplified by decreased skin elasticity, reduced barrier function, development of skin rhytids, epidermal and dermal thinning, and pigmentary changes.[18,19] Stem cells residing in various stem cell niches in the hair follicle, in interfollicular epidermis, and in sebaceous glands have been shown to play an important role in the maintenance of skin homeostasis.[20–22]

Our skin is the largest organ in our body and is responsible for many critical physiologic functions. It varies in thickness from 0.05 to 2 mm and is composed of 4 main layers. The outermost layer (stratum corneum) is 10 to 20 μm. There is a highly hydrophobic layer that consists of 10 to 15 layers of nonviable cells called corneocytes. These hydrated corneocytes serve as a protective barrier and are held together by multiple lipid bio-layers composed of fatty acids, cholesterol and cholesterol esters, and ceramides.[23–25] The epidermis is the second layer and is subdivided into the stratum lucidium, stratum granulosum, stratum spinosum, and stratum germinatevum (basale). The epidermis is composed of keratinocytes that are in various stages of differentiation. Keratinocytes comprise 95% of the dermis. Those in the stratum terminal type layer are often referred to as "basal cells." Although keratinocytes are the predominant epidermal cell, melanocytes, Merkel cells, Langerhans cells, dendritic T cells, and adipose cells also are present. In addition, multiple catabolic enzymes, such as proteases, nucleotides, esterases, phosphatases, and lipases, are present in the intracellular spaces. MSCs residing in the skin are responsible for cellular signaling that regulates keratinocyte differentiation and influences other cellular functions to regulate homeostasis.[26–28] The basement membrane is attached to the dermis and provides a physical boundary between the epithelium and the dermis. It is rich in extracellular matrix proteins and growth factors. The dermis is composed of sebaceous glands, nerves, blood vessels, and hair follicles, as well as adipose cells, mass cells, and infiltrating leukocytes.[29] The final layer is the subcutaneous layer (hypodermis), which is composed primarily of adipose cells, MSCs, blood vessels, and lymphatics.

Previously it was felt that the primary purpose of adipose tissue was to serve as a support structure and as a reservoir of energy in the form of triglycerides and as a storehouse for fat-soluble vitamins. However, numerous studies in recent years have demonstrated that adipose tissue provides significant influence on the cellular microenvironment by secretion of a wide range of bioactive factors with a diverse set of functions. Lipid metabolism and insulin sensitivity appeared to be influenced, as is the regulation of angiogenesis, immunomodulation, and inflammatory response. Adipose tissue secretory profile appears to influence tissue and organ homeostasis at the autocrine, paracrine, and endocrine levels.[30] Studies have revealed that they also appear to be involved in mediation and management of keratinocyte and fibroblast proliferation and migration to ensure epidermal and dermal repair.[21,31,32] Thus, adipose tissue–resident MSCs can be viewed as "endogenous factories" producing trophic mediators able to support all of the functional skin layers to ensure skin homeostasis, regulation, and repair.[11]

ASCs have been shown to secrete several growth factors: vascular endothelial growth factor (VEGF), hepatocyte growth factor, fibroblast growth factor 2, and insulin-like growth factor 1 (IGF-1). Travers and Spandau and their colleagues[33–36] have reported on the role of IGF-1 in potentially reducing the incidence of skin cancer via its effect on keratinocytes. Preliminary studies by the author indicate that IGF-1 may also play a role in reducing cutaneous rhytids.[37]

Gimble and colleagues[38,39] have shown that ASCs introduced into injured tissue results in secretion of cytokines and growth factors that stimulate recovery in a paracrine manner. Gimbel points out that ASCs modulate the "stem cell niche" of the host by stimulating the recruitment of endogenous cytokines themselves to the site of injury and promote stem cell differentiation along the required lineage pathway. It is theorized that ASCs could provide antioxidants, free radical scavengers, and chaperone/heat shock proteins at an ischemic site. Toxic substances released into the local cellular environment as a direct result of the injury would be removed, thus promoting cell recovery and survival. Thus, ASCs appear to play a significant, yet not clearly defined role in such diverse processes as skin cancer prevention, wound healing, and aesthetic enhancement of aging skin.

Dermatologic aging is influenced by intrinsic and external factors. Structural changes are a result of changes and alterations in biological molecules: proteins, glycosaminoglycan, and lipids.[40,41] With aging, the epidermis thins. This is caused by reduction in vascularity and hydration. The thickness of the epidermis is reduced approximately 6.4% each decade with an associated decrease in the number of mast cells and fibroblasts.[40,42,43] This reduction in total fibroblasts results in reduced production of collagen, elastin, glycosaminoglycans, and hyaluronic acid, which leads to thinning of the dermis.[44]

Various growth factors and cytokines influenced by stem cells have an impact on the aging process. Recent studies have shown interleukins and interleukin receptors in the skin to play an important role in the regulation of the inflammatory stage of wound healing and regeneration.[45–47] Additional studies have shown low doses of interleukins to have an antiaging effect.[48,49] IGF-1 and its binding proteins have also been shown to have an impact on aging. The ratio between IGF-1 and insulin growth factor binding protein 3 has been associated with facial aging and skin wrinkling by means of its influence on collagen biosynthesis.[50] In addition, dermal adipocytes have been shown to secrete adipo-cytokines such as adiponectin and leptin, which results in increased production of hyaluronic acid and collagen by human dermal fibroblasts, promoting wound healing in the skin.[51,52]

Some clinicians have simply injected stem cells into the skin as a therapeutic modality to promote wound healing, tissue restoration, and skin rejuvenation. However, work by Zhu and colleagues[53,54] suggests that ASCs injected into the soft tissue or into a defect will not alone produce soft tissue fill. They advocate using a tissue-engineering approach, combining cells stimulated with certain chemical compounds and placed into a matrix or scaffold to "manufacture" an implantable neoadipose construct. In general, fillers currently on the market have not been successful in supporting an engineered tissue replacement therapy for defect repair or tissue restoration. Identifying the appropriate filler in combination with stem cells could provide an optimized microenvironment in which to create an engineered tissue that can be used as a semipermanent filler material.

Moseley and colleagues[55] noted that biomaterials can serve as a scaffold support or matrix for infiltrating cells in the wound-healing process. These biomaterials have been combined with adipocyte precursors or dermal fibroblasts to produce engineered constructs for volume augmentation. The limiting factor in this process appears to be the rapidity and extent of neovascularization of the construct. It may take as long as 5 days for blood vessels from adjacent tissue to infiltrate into the construct and provide appropriate vascularization. This time delay can result in tissue necrosis and cell death.

Investigators have studied multiple potential scaffolds combined with cells to evaluate their utility for soft tissue treatment. Altman and colleagues[56] reported that MRI studies revealed a consistent and stable volume fill by ASCs and non–animal-stabilized hyaluronic acid at 3 weeks. ASCs actively incorporated into the hyaluronic acid fill and showed an organized fibrovascular network at 3 weeks. They concluded that the combination of ASCs and non–animal-stabilized hyaluronic acid shows promise as a vehicle with which to achieve lasting volume fill in reconstructive surgical soft tissue augmentation.

In another study, Stillaert and colleagues[57] compared the hyaluronic acid sponge, HYAFF 11, with collagen sponges augmented with adipose precursor cells. HYAFF 11 was noted to be superior to collagen in supporting the differentiation and expansion of adipose precursor cells.

Chung and colleagues[58] reported on using hyaluronic acid–immobilized porous biodegradable microspheres for producing injectable MSC aggregates for adipose tissue regeneration. They reported that hyaluronic acid–immobilized microspheres significantly enhanced cell differentiation and tissue regeneration when implanted in vivo, compared with unmodified porous microspheres. Their studies showed that adipose tissue–derived MSC cellular aggregates prepared by using porous microspheres could be delivered in an injectable manner into the body and could have great therapeutic potential for soft tissue augmentation and reconstruction.

Studies by Woo and colleagues[59] demonstrated that beta-glucan and porous poly-lactide-co-glycoside (PLGA) membranes containing beta-glucans enhanced the cellular proliferation of adult human dermal fibroblasts and ASCs. Their studies suggest that beta-glucan and porous PLGA membranes containing beta-glucan may be useful as a material for enhancing wound healing.

Deployment of stem cells with adipocytes serving as a carrier has increased in popularity. Tholpady and colleagues[60] reported using autologous fat as a matrix and supplemented the transplant with ASCs. They noted that this resulted in long-term (more than 1 year) soft tissue volume restoration in a patient with soft tissue involution on the ulnar aspect of one hand.[60] Zhu, Yoshimura and others have published on breast augmentation using stem cell–enhanced adipocyte transfer and have noted 60% increased fat survival as compared with 35% with fat only.[61] In the Yoshimura study, 40 patients had 270 mL injected into each breast with 60% to 80% of breast fat remaining after 2 years.[1]

ACQUISITION, CULTURE, AND EXPANSION OF ADIPOSE-DERIVED STEM CELLS

Following the identification in 2006 of adipose tissue as a rich source of adult MSCs and subsequent realization of their regenerative potential and wound-healing properties, there has been a stimulation in its use in a variety of clinical applications.[62–65] ASCs are typically obtained from lipo-aspirate, which is harvested via tumescent abdominal liposuction techniques or by surgical resection of adipose tissue that is then diced into the smaller segments for processing.[66] The adipose tissue, harvested either via lipo-aspiration or direct excision method, undergoes further processing using either enzymatic digestion[67,68] or via mechanical cell separation.[64,69] Although there is extensive use of adipose tissue in clinical applications, there is no single standard protocol available for isolation and preparation of adipose tissue.[11] However, most isolation protocols consist of 4 basic steps: (1) washing

lipo-aspirate, (2) collagenase enzyme processing, (3) centrifugation, and (4) removal of red blood cells. This process results in the production of a small pellet that is a heterogeneous collection of cells, approximately 5% of which are stem cells. Based on laboratory experience, a volume of 500 mL of lipo-aspirate will provide nearly 1×10^9 ASCs. This pellet is termed the "stromal vascular fraction" (SVF). Plating out the pellet produces adipose-derived MSCs.

Isolation of ASCs is an extremely complex process that involves specialized equipment and specialized reagents, and requires compliance with good manufacturing practices (GMP)/good clinical practices (GCP) practice guidelines. The following are examples of procedures for isolation and processing of ASCs via SVF.[1]

The process typically can take more than 8 hours. However, Francis and colleagues[70] reported on a technique for isolating viable populations of MSCs from lipo-aspirate fractions within 30 minutes. Reducing acquisition time of ASCs can have a significant positive impact on their use in tissue engineering and regenerative medicine.

A syringe filled with adipose tissue harvested by lipo-aspirate technique or by direct excision would be placed in a sterile blood baguette and washed 3 times with sterile Dulbecco's phosphate-buffered saline to eliminate erythrocytes. The adipose tissue is then transferred to 60-mL sterile centrifuge containers followed by addition of a collagenase enzyme to disrupt the fibrous tissue (0.3 mg/mL Liberase Blendzyme 1 using a 1:1 volume ratio).

A shaker bath at 37°C. could be used for 30 minutes until a milky solution is produced or centrifuge containers could be sealed and placed in the water bath for 1 hour, then centrifuged for 7 minutes at 300g. During centrifugation, the stromal cells form a pellet at the bottom of the container, while the adipocyte layer and debris remain suspended.

The top layer is removed. The next layer is a collagenase solution. The "pellet" is at the bottom. The pellet is a heterogeneous collection of cells, approximately 5% of which are stem cells. The pellet is also termed the SVF. Plating out the pellet produces MSCs.

Protocols for isolation of ASCs from adipose tissue using enzymatic digestion have been broadly applied by many researchers. In an alternative isolation technique, liposuction aspirate or finely minced adipose tissue is washed extensively with sterile phosphate-buffered saline to remove blood cells, saline, and local anesthetics. Extracellular matrix is digested with 0.075% collagenase at 37°C for 30 minutes to release the cellular fraction. Collagenase is inactivated with an equal volume of

Dulbecco modified Eagle medium (DMEM) containing 10% fetal bovine serum (FBS). The infranatant is centrifuged at 250g for 10 minutes to obtain a high-density cell pellet. The pellet is resuspended in DMEM and 10% FBS and plated in 100-mm tissue culture dishes at a density of 1 × 10^6 cells per plate. These cells are maintained in control medium (DMEM supplemented with 10% FBS and 1% antibiotic/antimycotic) at 37°C and 5% CO_2. Attached cells exhibit a fibroblastlike appearance and the potential to differentiate into adipogenic, osteogenic, chondrogenic, myogenic, and neurogenic lineages under the appropriate culture conditions.[12]

ASC cultures under standard conditions exhibit an average population doubling time of 60 hours. The age of the donor, the type of adipose tissue (white or brown adipose tissue), the type of surgical procedure for preparing the specimen, culturing conditions, plating density, and media formulations all can impact the rate of tissue growth.

Stromal Vascular Fraction

SVF contains not only ASCs, but also a mixed composition of cells which includes preadipocytes, adipocytes, macrophages, endothelial progenitor cells and growth factors.[9,71] SVF has been shown to be a rich source of growth factors such as platelet-derived growth factor (PDGF)-BB, VEGF, IGF-1, and basic fibroblast growth factor.[72]

Because of significant differences in protocols for harvesting, processing, and techniques for deployment of cells (injection techniques), it is extremely difficult to make comparisons of outcomes of clinical therapies.[73] A recent review comparing isolation techniques and processing protocols found no significant differences and therapeutic benefits dependent on preoperative site preparation, adipose tissue harvesting techniques, centrifugation speed, or cannula size for harvesting.[74] However, additional studies and reviews are needed to substantiate these conclusions.

Culturing of Adipose-Derived Stem Cells

ASCs can be expanded via culturing techniques. This can result in a homogeneous ASC population that expresses surface markers similar to bone marrow MSCs, CD29, CV44, CD73, CD90, and CD105, while being negative for hematopoietic lineage markers CD 31, CD34, and CD45.[2] Multiple studies have been conducted regarding secretory properties, cell surface expression markers, multipotent potential, and immunomodulatory properties of ASCs and bone marrow–derived MSCs. These studies have concluded that secretory properties are similar for both ASCs and bone marrow–derived MSCs.[20,30,75–77]

Various clinical studies have demonstrated that ASCs accelerate wound closure, reduce scarring, promote collagen synthesis, promote angiogenesis, and improve wound tensile strength.[78] ASCs maintained in platelet-rich plasma (PRP)-containing media have been shown to have a stimulatory effect on the proliferation and migration of dermal fibroblasts and keratinocytes.[63,79,80] This cellular influence of ASCs is thought to be a result of a double paracrine loop that exemplifies the intricate relationships between ASCs in the various cellular components of the dermis and epidermis that are involved in tissue homeostasis.[10,20,26,81]

Although studies have shown a therapeutic effect from the use of ASC transplants or conditioned media, there is no reliable information regarding the impact donor age has regarding ASC regenerative or wound-healing potential. Conflicting data are available concerning the effects of donor age on ASC function.[30,82,83] However, Kato and colleagues[32] recently reported data that showed that, although the treatment with adult bone marrow–derived MSCs or ASCs in cutaneous wounds facilitated wound healing and regeneration, both of these therapies were negatively impacted by advanced stem cell donor age.

It is important to note that prolonged ex vivo culturing of ASCs can result in significant and measurable changes due to the process of replicative senescence.[30,82,84] This is manifested by loss of control of chromatin organization and activates a persistent DNA damage response that causes robust changes in transcriptional activity.[85,86] These changes result in both reduction of differentiation potential of ASCs and changes in their secretory profile, which impacts paracrine function and immunomodulation.[87,88] Gaur and colleagues[11,87,88] theorized that the role of senescence in aging of the adult stem cells is tightly linked to tissue maintenance and homeostasis and often viewed as an irreversible barrier to immobilization and tumorigenesis under the assumption that cellular senescence evolved to suppress tumorigenesis.

CLINICAL STUDIES REGARDING ADIPOSE-DERIVED STEM CELLS AND ASSOCIATED GROWTH FACTORS AND CYTOKINE AND CURRENT THERAPEUTIC APPLICATIONS

In recent years, a multitude of studies have demonstrated that MSCs have antiaging effects.

Song and colleagues[89] investigated the effects of ASCs on human dermal fibroblasts that were damaged through photoaging due to UVB irradiation. Photo-damaged human fibroblasts showed greater proliferation rates in the presence of ASCs and their secreted growth factors and cytokines. Metalloproteinase (MMP-1) is a known initiator of photodamage in the skin and is typically increased in fibroblasts after UV irradiation. P16 is a gene that controls the cell cycle and acts as a marker of cellular senescence or aging. ASCs reversed damage in photoaged fibroblasts. ASCs reduced the number of apoptotic cells and shifted the cell cycles from necrosis to late to early apoptosis. The study by Song and colleagues[89] concluded that ASCs mediate their antiaging effects through a paracrine function on fibroblasts and can reverse damage in photoaged fibroblasts at both the cell cycle and genetic levels.

Park and colleagues[90] previously demonstrated that ASCs stimulate collagen synthesis and migration of fibroblasts during wound healing. In this study, they verified the mechanisms of action and effects of ASCs on skin aging. Secretory factors of ASCs were investigated, and many growth factors were identified. ASC therapy caused increased dermal thickening and collagen production. In a case study, ASCs were injected intradermally (2 successive injections at 2-week intervals). After 2 months, improved skin texture and increased dermal thickness were documented. Park and colleagues[90] concluded that ASCs produce useful growth factors, increase collagen production, and reverse skin aging.

Antiaging of the skin is mediated by a combination of the effects of time (intrinsic aging) and environmental factors (extrinsic aging) on cellular and extracellular infrastructure. These are 2 independent, clinically and biologically distinct, processes that affect the skin structure and function simultaneously. Growing evidence now suggests that the 2 aging processes have converging biochemical and molecular pathways that lead to photoaging of skin. The common mechanisms of the 2 aging processes may provide several unique opportunities to develop antiaging therapies. Recent advances in understanding the role of endogenous growth factors in the aging process provide one such opportunity to develop topical antiaging products.[91]

The use of growth factors and cytokines for skin rejuvenation and reversal of photoaging is emerging as a novel antiaging treatment. Kim and colleagues[92] showed that radio-frequency created, microporated skin, actually created micro-channels for the topical application of growth factors. One month after 3 treatment sessions, histologic studies demonstrated increase in both dermal thickness and dermal collagen. Waibel and colleagues[93–97] recently reported similar finds and favorable results modifying cutaneous scaring by using lasers to recreate micro-channels to facilitate cutaneous absorption of topically applied stem cells and stem cell–derived growth factors.

Park and colleagues reported compelling results in a large-scale study for ASC protein extract applied transdermally. Providing growth factors and cytokines to cells responsible for extracellular matrix production appeared to stimulate rejuvenation of aging skin.[98]

Brohem and colleagues[99] compared fibroblasts with MSCs derived from bone marrow, skin, and adipose tissue to assess the differentiation potential of fibroblasts. Their studies showed that fibroblasts expressed the same cell immunophenotypic markers as stem cells and were able to differentiate into the 3 cell lineages: adipocytes, osteocytes, and chondrocytes.

Fabi and Sundaram[100] noted growth factors and cytokines control skin growth, proliferation, and differentiation by means of intercellular and intracellular signaling pathways. They noted striking parallels between the pathways involved in skin wound healing and photoaging of skin. They noted that topical application of growth factors and injection of growth factors contained in an autologous PRP had a positive effect on skin regeneration and rejuvenation. They noted that growth factors associated with stem cell proteins secreted by human dermal fibroblasts under hypoxic stress accelerated skin healing after laser resurfacing. They also noted that platelet-rich fibrin matrix facilitated skin rejuvenation.

Lee and colleagues[101] reported on efficacy of micro-needling plus human stem cell conditioned medium for skin rejuvenation in a randomized controlled blinded, split-face study in 25 women. Human ESC conditioned medium was applied topically with enhanced dermal presentation achieved by using a 0.25-mm micro-needle roller. Treatment sessions were repeated at 2-week intervals. Improvement was noted with both pigmentation and wrinkles. Their conclusion was that secretory factors of endothelial precursor cells differentiated from human ESCs improved the signs of skin aging. Sasaki[102,103] recently reported similar findings with micro-needling.

Hussain and colleagues[104] reported on ultrastructural changes after the use of human growth factors and cytokine skin cream as a treatment for skin rejuvenation. They noted clinical, histologic, and ultrastructural changes observed after 6 months of application of a topical skin cream containing human growth factors and cytokines applied twice daily for 6 months. Clinical appearance and periorbital wrinkles improved by 33% and perioral wrinkling by 25%. Histologic evaluation indicated moderate changes in epidermal thickness as well as increased fibroblast density in the superficial dermis. Electron microscopy showed ultrastructural changes consistent with new collagen formation. Their study collaborates previous studies by other researchers showing that topical application of growth factors and cytokines is beneficial in reducing signs of facial skin aging.

Sundaram and colleagues[105] showed topically applied physiologically balanced growth factors, in spite of large molecular weight, showed evidence suggesting that a small fraction of topically applied growth factors secreted by human fibroblasts grown in conditions resembling the physiologic condition of the dermis and in high concentrations and in a stable formula penetrates into the deeper dermis and exhibits a physiologic effect. Clinical studies showed that topical application of a product with high concentrations of physiologically balanced mixture growth factors appears to reduce signs of skin aging.

Several cosmeceutical products containing either a single human growth factor or a combination of multiple human growth factors and cytokines are currently being marketed for skin rejuvenation. Clinical results for some of these products show that human growth factors, when applied topically, appear to provide beneficial effects in reducing the signs of facial aging. Mehta and Fitzpatrick[91] and Fitzpatrick and Rostan[106] reported on a proprietary mixture of growth factors and cytokines secreted by cultured neonatal human dermal fibroblasts. Patients were treated twice daily for 60 days. Results showed a 12% reduction in periorbital wrinkling after 60 days. Histologic studies showed 37% increase in Grenz-zone collagen and a 30% increase in dermal thickness.

Hydrophilic molecules larger than 500-Da molecular weight have very little penetration through stratum corneum. Growth factors and cytokines are large hydrophilic molecules, more than 15,000 Da molecular weight and are very unlikely to penetrate through the epidermis in amounts able to produce pharmacologic effects. Despite this fact, results of clinical studies by Fitzpatrick and others[91,106] show that topical application of these macro molecules may produce clinical benefits. The primary mechanism by which the growth factors and cytokines can potentially exert their effect on the dermal matrix is by penetration through hair follicles, sweat glands, or compromised skin, followed by interaction with

cells in the dermis, such as keratinocytes, to produce signaling cytokines that affect cells (such as fibroblasts) that are deeper in the dermis. Skin may contain small imperfections resulting from dryness, scratching, or use of products containing irritating chemicals that may allow small amounts of these macro molecules to penetrate into the viable portions of the epidermis. Addition of lipophilic penetration enhancers or barrier-alternating peptides, may also increase penetration of these proteins through intact skin. Recent studies have shown that vaccines can exert immunologic response when applied topically. This probably results from penetration of a very small amount of protein through intact skin. Similar extent of penetration also may be sufficient for topically applied growth factors to produce an effect on epidermal cells. Epidermal-dermal communications appear to mediate the effects of topically applied growth factors and cytokines. Evidence strongly suggests the presence of a double paracrine loop in which keratinocytes stimulate fibroblasts to synthesize growth factors, that in turn stimulate keratinocyte proliferation, which results in amplification of the initial effect of topical growth factors. Keratinocytes have surface receptors for many growth factors and cytokines, some of which are present in cosmetic products. Penetration of small amounts of these molecules into the viable portion of the epidermis after topical application can induce keratinocytes to produce growth factors (PDGF, interleukin-1, transforming growth factor [TGF]-alpha, and TGF-beta) that have been shown to exert a paracrine effect on proliferation and activation of dermal fibroblasts, which leads to regeneration and remodeling of the dermal extracellular matrix. Although it is unclear how large proteins, such as growth factors, are able to penetrate the skin and become pharmacologically effective, early objective clinical studies and subjective observations indicate that these cosmeceutical products may potentially reduce signs of facial aging.

SKIN REGENERATION AND WOUND HEALING

Pitanguy and colleagues have pointed out that restoring skin would require extensive self-renewing stem cells. This is because skin is characterized by an extensive self-renewal process. They noted that progenitor cells represented in a keratinocyte culture would be capable of generating epidermal grafts.[107] The basal layer contains 2 types of proliferative keratinocytes: stem cells, which have unlimited self-renewal capacity, and transit amplifying cells, "daughters" of stem cells that will terminally differentiate after a few rounds of division. Cells for a skin substitute can be derived from local, systemic, and progenitor cell populations. Fibroblasts, keratinocytes, melanocytes, adipocytes, and hair follicle cells can be sourced locally and could be used for skin tissue engineering. Systemic cells are populations of cells that reside in the blood or bone marrow (such as fibrocytes) and are known to play an important role in skin wound healing. Progenitor cells are located in stem cell niches, such as the hair follicle, and also reside in the bone marrow.[108]

Garcia-Olmo and colleagues[109] reported on using ASCs to treat nonhealing fistula tracts in patients with Crohn disease. Following liposuction, stem cells were isolated and expanded in culture. These ASCs were then deployed into the fistula tracts of patients with Crohn disease. A 75% closure rate was noted.[47] Garcia-Olmo and colleagues[109] then came back and used the pellet (the SVF) that was obtained at the time of surgery. When this was injected in the fistulous tract, they obtained a 25% fistula closure rate. Thus, in this study, the cultured (expanded) MSCs were 3 times as effective in promoting wound healing in contaminated wounds as were the SVFs. They concluded that cultured or manipulated stem cells secrete more growth factors or more specific cytokines to positively influence wound healing.

Autologous ASCs have been used for the regenerative treatment of traumatic calvarial bone defects using autologous cancellous iliac bone in combination with autologous stem cells and fibrin glue. Postoperative computed tomography (CT) studies have demonstrated new bone formation with good clinical results in a limited number of cases.[110]

STEM CELL AUGMENTATION OF ADIPOSE TISSUE GRAFTS: CELL-ASSISTED LIPOMA TRANSFER

Soft tissue defects represent a reconstructive challenge. Rubin and Marra[111] reported in 2011 that more than 5.6 million procedures were performed in the United States regarding this problem. Although most cases arise from tumor extraction and the sequelae of adjunctive radiation therapy, defects of soft tissue occur from congenital abnormalities, following trauma, and are being addressed with volumization procedures for aesthetic concerns.

In cell-assisted lipo–transfer (CAL), ASCs are harvested from lipo-aspirate and are used to supplement fat grafts to enhance reconstruction of facial asymmetries, post-cancer radiation effects, traumatic wounds, and aesthetic concerns.[112]

Yoshimura noted that aspirated fat was relatively stem cell–deficient and the mechanical disruption of the adipose tissue during liposuction was thought to contribute to this loss of stem cells. Yoshimura and colleagues[110,114] in 2008 noted improved graft retention with the supplementation of fat cells with additional adipose stem cells. Animal studies by Matsumoto and colleagues[113] in 2006 with subcutaneous implantation of human CAL fat grafts into immunodeficient mice demonstrated 35% increased volume retention when compared with conventional lipo transfer. Tanikawa and colleagues[115] in 2013 conducted a randomized study on patients with cranial facial microsomia. CAL was found to enhance fat volume retention compared with supplemental fat grafts. CT scans 6 months after grafting revealed 80% survival among patients with CAL fat grafts compared with 54% for controls, suggesting this to be an effective treatment modality for facial recontouring. Showing similar clinical support for this technique, Kolle and colleagues[116] in 2013 performed a blinded, placebo-controlled trial in which 30-mL fat grafts with and without the addition of 20 million expanded ASCs per milliliter of fat were injected into the upper arm. After 4 months, CAL fat grafts exhibited a 64.6% increased volume. Subsequent clinical and preclinical trials by Garza and colleagues[117] (2014), Tanikawa and colleagues[115] (2013), Yoshimura[114] (2008) and others have confirmed enhanced fat graft retention when enriched with ASCs.[118]

Ischemia is inherent in the process of grafting tissue. Suga and colleagues[119] in 2010 showed that ASCs appeared to be relatively resistant to hypoxic conditions and contribute to adipose tissue regeneration. There is a notion that ASCs may undergo adipogenic differentiation and assist in regeneration of fat.[120] However, more recent studies Garza and colleagues[117] in 2014, have suggested only transient retention of supplemental ASCs within fat grafts, and that the regions of necrosis are ultimately replaced by recipient site–derived adipocytes.[118,121,122] Both of these observations argue against the substantial contribution of ASCs to mature adipocyte tissue. Alternatively, adipose tissue is known to be rich in microvasculature and ASCs that reside around capillaries and vessels have been shown to be capable of in vitro differentiation into the vascular endothelial cells.[123]

Matsumoto and colleagues[113] performed studies using labeled ASCs implanted with fat and showed that they subsequently stained positive for von Willebrand factor, suggesting their ability to differentiate into vascular endothelial cells and contribute to vasculogenesis in the acute phase following transplantation. However, recent studies by Garza and colleagues[117] and Dong (2015) argue against a direct role of ASCs in early revascularization. Nevertheless, ASCs likely exhibit a paracrine effect and have been shown to release androgenic growth factors. Zhu and colleagues[53] reported high levels of expression in ASCs of multiple proandrogenic growth factors and noted increased capillary density within fat grafts supplemented with ASCs. Garza and colleagues[117] in studies retrieved supplemental ASCs following fat grafting and noted significant upregulation of angiogenic gene expression. All of these studies support a paracrine role for ASCs, promoting early revascularization of ischemic fat grafts to reduce adipocyte apoptosis and enhance long-term retention.

The critical question is how many cells are necessary to affect a meaningful (positive) change in fat graft retention. Historically, most studies report using a 1:1 approach, using one-half of the harvested specimen for the actual adipose tissue graft and processing the other half to obtain the material to serve as "supplement" for the graft.[114,115,124]

Paik and colleagues[125] reported performing titration studies regarding the number of ASCs added to autologous human fat and found that 1 $\times$ 10^5 supplemental cells per 200 mL fat graft produced the greatest improvement in volume retention and vascularity. Interestingly, significantly greater numbers of supplemental ASCs resulted in decreased fat graft retention, thought to be secondary to cell-cell competition between ASCs and fat graft adipocytes for the scarce resources in the hypoxic environment.

CURRENT TRENDS FOR CLINICAL RESEARCH AND QUESTIONS THAT REMAIN TO BE ANSWERED

There is functional heterogeneity among ASCs. Whether these differences in ASC behavior are due to the actions of different ASC subpopulations or the effects of the tissue microenvironment on cell activity remains unknown. ASCs are heterogeneous with subpopulations of both proangiogenic and proadipogenic ASCs. In addition, Levi and colleagues[126–128] have pointed out that there may also be pro-osteogenic fractions.[129–131] Thus, differences in the physical microenvironment of ASCs may account for the lack of adipogenic signaling observed in supplemental ASCs in CAL. These cells are simply mixed in solution with lipo-aspirate. Ongoing research by Memon and colleagues,[132] Sivan and colleagues,[133,134] continues to investigate the use of artificial niches to direct differentiation of ASCs into keratinocytes,

cardio-myocytes, osteoblasts, and other cell types.[135]

There are 4 key questions that future research must answer for ASCs to become uniformly accepted treatment modalities:

1. What subpopulations of ASCs exist?

   ASCs prepared from human liposuction aspirate from different studies exhibit differences in purity and molecular phenotype. Many studies show that cell preparations likely contain heterogeneous populations of cells, which makes it uncertain whether the ASCs themselves are actually responsible for the observed effects.

2. What are the parameters that define the ASC niche?

3. What potential protumorigenic and antitumorigenic properties of ASCs can best be titrated to maximize the potential of using ASCs in the setting of reconstructive and aesthetic surgery?

   Immunologic and angiogenic properties of ASCs raises questions of the relationship of the cells with promoting cancer. There are several contrary studies that have been published, some reports demonstrating that ASCs could promote tumor growth. Conversely, other studies support that ASCs can have a tumor suppressive affect.

   In 2005, a priority report was published in the journal *Cancer Research* from scientists in Spain and the United Kingdom as the first report of spontaneous malignant transformation of human adult stem cells, supporting the hypothesis of cancer stem cell origin. They noted that although there were clinical trials that reported the safety of human adult stem cells, showing them to be highly resistant to malignant transformation, there were clear similarities between stem cells and cancer stem cell genetic makeup. They noted that although cells could be managed safely during the standard ex vivo expansion of 6 to 8 weeks, human MSCs could undergo spontaneous malignant transformation following long-term in vitro culture of 4 to 5 months. This report obviously garnered significant attention, with the result that others were unable to duplicate the reported findings. The authors and the journal subsequently retracted the paper in 2010.[136]

   Breast cancer: The journal *Stem Cell International* (2015)[137] reported on a review of breast cancer and stem cells. Their conclusion was that most experimental studies tend to support the propensity of MSCs and ASCs in promoting growth and progression and metastatic spread of residual or de novo breast cancer after resection. In contrast, however, only a few clinical case series and trials actually reflected this. Overall, they felt that most the studies did not support using autologous stem cell–enhanced grafts, whereas they felt that whole fat grafting appeared to be safe in most circumstances.

Although mesenchymal stromal cells represent a heterogeneous population of multipotent cells with beneficial properties for regenerative processes and with therapeutic benefit for patients being demonstrated in a wide range of severe pathologic conditions, mesenchymal stromal cell therapy also may be associated with adverse effects, such as an increased recurrence rate for hematologic malignancies.[138]

Human mesenchymal stromal cells were shown to be nontumorigenic. However, there have been reports of their capability to modulate the tumor microenvironment, thus having an impact on tumor behavior. There is increasing evidence that mesenchymal stromal cells might play a role in tumor pathogenesis and progression. Kucerova and colleagues[139] demonstrated the tumor-promoting effect of adipose tissue–derived mesenchymal stromal cells on human melanoma A375 cells.

Rubio and colleagues[136] reported that human ASCs can undergo malignant transformation with prolonged passaging over more than 4 months. Some feel that this may indicate that freshly isolated ASCs could possibly be a safer and a more practical source than cultured ASCs for clinical use.

Mesenchymal stromal cells produce cytokines and can give rise to endothelial-like cells contributing to tumor vascular formation. Mesenchymal stromal cells were noted to have the capability to differentiate into carcinoma-associated fibroblasts when under the influence of tumor-cell produced soluble factors. Manipulated human mesenchymal stromal cells were shown to have increased metastatic potential for breast cancer cells rather than significant tumor growth.[140,141]

4. What are the ongoing concerns regarding ASCs in the clinical setting?

RESEARCH TRENDS AND FOOD AND DRUG ADMINISTRATION OVERSIGHT

In February 2014, the Food and Drug Administration (FDA) Commissioner, the FDA Center for Biologics and Evaluation Research, and the Office of Cellular, Tissue and Gene Therapy published the FDA perspective on mesenchymal stromal cell (MSC)-based clinical trials.[142] There are 4 basic parameters that the FDA feels influence the final stem cell product: FBS, atmospheric oxygen, cryopreservation, and cell banking. In the past decade there has been a 300% increase in the number of Investigational New Drug trials regarding MSCs. Most of these clinical trials (73% in 2012) were with allogeneic donors. Bone morrow was the leading source for stem cells in the United States, accounting for 55% of cases in 2013. This is in contrast to worldwide data that shows bone marrow–derived stem cells comprising fewer than half of all studies. Adipose tissue was the third most common stem cell source. However, it should be noted that there was a threefold increase in adipose tissue studies from 2011 to 2012. More than 80% of the trials used stem cells cultured in FBS, with the average concentration being 10%. It is important to point out that approximately 11% of the population has a bovine-related allergy and there has been a move away from these products. However, they still comprise a significant majority of the current stem cell studies. There has been considerable discussion in the medical literature, advocated by Yoshumoro[114] and others, regarding increased activity of stem cells when cultured in a hypoxic environment. However, 90% of US studies are using atmospheric oxygen. Cryopreservation is used by 80% to store and transport the final product, with the product being thawed within a few hours of patient infusion. Most protocols call for post-thaw cell viability to exceed 70%. Thirty-five percent of studies use cell banking, meaning that they bank the sample and expand the cell culture through multiple passages. Cardiovascular was the leading area for clinical stem cell trials followed by neurologic and then orthopedics. Although multiple routes of administration are used, more than 50% of the clinical trials call for the stem cells to be administered intravenously. Currently, 7 phenotypic cell markers are commonly used to monitor stem cells. However, the FDA is encouraging expanding this number, pointing out that markers can predict potential therapeutic benefits.

Gir and colleagues[143] conducted a review of the literature regarding the basic science evidence of ongoing clinical trials involving the use of ASCs in regenerative medicine. Only 33 clinical trial studies based on ASC therapy were identified. Most studies were performed in Spain and in Korea, with only 3 trials in the United States. In all published cases, there were no major adverse events reported and results regarding soft tissue augmentation and wound healing were noted to be very encouraging. The investigators noted that there were no standards or protocols for ASC use and that further basic science experimental studies with standardized protocols and larger, randomized controlled trials were called for.

To provide a more contemporary assessment of current clinical studies, a review of clinicaltrials.gov registered studies as of April 30, 2016, was conducted. Regarding ASCs or bone marrow–derived stem cells, a total of 164 studies were registered. Only 1 study was noted in the hair restoration area and 4 studies were noted pertaining to photoaging and wound healing. A review of clinical studies dealing with hair was conducted. Eleven studies dealing in some degree with hair growth or hair stimulation were noted. Most studies were using PRP. The others studies used adipose tissue, mainly adipose-derived SVF. A review of clinical studies dealing with photoaging was conducted. Seven studies were noted that dealt with photoaging. One study used bone marrow–derived stem cells to be administered intravenously for photoaging. One study used ASCs plus hyaluronic acid as a dermal filler. Other photoaging studies were mainly using PRP. Two studies used adipose tissue–derived SVF plus fat for enhanced fat graft viability.

STATUS OF FOOD AND DRUG ADMINISTRATION OVERSIGHT AND REGULATIONS: CELLULAR AND TISSUE THERAPIES

Scientific and technological advances in stem cell biology and tissue engineering have led to the increased use of human cells and tissues for the treatment of various diseases, injuries, and aesthetic concerns. The regulatory environment for cell and tissue therapy products is rapidly evolving, with various drug regulatory agencies in many countries implementing regulatory controls in the past several years. In the United States, that responsibility is under the auspices of the FDA and more specifically, the Center for Biologics Evaluation and Research (CBER).[144,145]

In the United States, stem cells are considered source material and fall under FDA Human Cells, Tissues, and Cellular and Tissue-Based Products (HCT/Ps) regulation for transplantable tissues and are regulated by the FDA CBER, and the Office of Cellular, Tissue and Gene Therapy. In general, the FDA has 5 major concerns relating to this area: (1) transmission of communicable disease, (2) processing control to prevent contamination and preserve product integrity and function, (3) clinical safety and efficacy, (4) promotional claims and labeling, and (5) how best to monitor and educate industry.

HCT/Ps are under the jurisdiction of the FDA for the regulation of transplantable tissues. When human tissues serve as "source material," the cellular products fall under the auspices of the FDA (Title 21: Food and Drugs; Chapter I - Food and Drug Administration; Subchapter L Regulations–Section 1271.3–human cells, tissues, and cellular in tissue-based products). Two specific sections are applicable to HCT/Ps. Section 361 regulates tissues (such as adipose tissue) and notes them to be exempt from regulation as HCT/Ps biological drugs if

1. cells or cellular material are "minimally manipulated"
2. cells or cellular material are not combined with any other agent (except water, crystalloids, or sterilizing, preserving, or storage agents are permitted)
3. cells or cellular material are for homologous use in the same individual ("Homologous use" is defined as the repair, reconstruction, replacement, or supplementation of a recipient's cells or tissues with an HCT/P that performs the same basic function or functions in the recipient as in the donor.)
4. cells or cellular material are collected and delivered at the "same surgical setting"

Section 351 applies to all other tissues, and processes are strictly regulated by the FDA. Cell culturing (expansion) would fall into this category, as would tissues that are more than minimally manipulated; tissues for uses not "homologous"; and when there are "additives" used in the preparation or extraction of the cells or tissues. In such cases, these "cellular products" are subject to the regulations for high-risk HCT/Ps, which include requiring the filing of a biologics license application; requesting permission from the FDA before proceeding to FDA-supervised clinical trials; and obtaining FDA approval before marketing the cellular therapy to the public. For example, harvesting autologous adipose tissue, extracting the stem cells by enzymatic digestion followed by centrifugation, and injecting the cells into nonfatty tissues (such as a joint, the heart, retina, or brain) would be considered a nonhomologous use of highly manipulated cellular materials. In this example, the FDA would consider the cellular materials to be biologic drugs, regulated under Section 351.

In response to the 21st Century Cures Act passed by Congress in November 2017, the FDA's CBER released its new guidelines for regenerative medicine. They included implementing a program designated as Regenerative Medicine Advanced Therapy. This program is available for certain cell therapies, therapeutic tissue engineering products, and certain combined products and closely mirrors accelerated pathways available for investigative drugs designed to meet serious unmet medical needs. The FDA also noted that, in an effort to modernize its regulatory framework to facilitate these scientific advances, they would consider real-world evidence of safety and efficacy, as opposed to strict requirements for such data to be drawn from prospective, randomized clinical trials.

At this time, the FDA also released guidance documents clarifying its intention to regulate manipulated cellular materials as biologic drugs. They clarified that "same surgical procedure" exemption extended only to rinsing, cleansing, sizing, and shaping of cells or tissue biomaterials. They also defined "minimal manipulation" as being processes that do not alter cells' structure or biological properties and "nonhomologous use" as functions different from those ordinarily exhibited by the same cells in vivo.

In recent years, there has been a plethora of stem cell clinics that have evolved. Some have been focused on primarily aesthetic concerns, whereas others have proactively marketed unproven stem cell "cures" for an extraordinary array of medical conditions. For this reason, there have been calls from many sectors for the FDA to increase its regulatory authority regarding stem cell therapies.

The FDA has taken some enforcement action in the adipose stem cell space. The November 2017 guidance documents could also be used by state attorneys general to stop stem cell clinics. More severe would be the impact on the plaintiffs' bar. Plaintiff attorneys could use final guidance documents as the basis to bring claims (even class actions) against stem cell clinics operating outside of an Investigation New Drug Study. Offering stem cell therapies that do not comply with FDA regulations could also void professional liability insurance coverage. In short, the potential implications flowing from the FDA's final guidance documents could have major impacts for physicians using stem cell therapies for aesthetic purposes.

There are 4 key areas that the FDA feels must have validation for future therapeutic uses of stem cells to be permitted: (1) Safety: must have disease screening of all donors and also ensure any agents used in manufacturing process have no deleterious effects. (2) Potency: must have validation assays to ensure consistency of processes and reactive agents so know the resultant reactions are reproducible. (3) Purity: look at flow cytometry and genetic analysis, want to be sure all cells are human (culture has not become contaminated and essentially that the cells are the type of cells that you think they are). If stem cell cultures are highly expanded, karyotyping is important to be sure there are no mutations. Typically, one would perform 3 passages: any pluripotent cells would have been removed in the process and you would be left with only multipotent cells (safer). (4) Efficacy: which is essentially outcome measurement.

There have been 2 main problems hampering stem cell therapy: (1) need to expand cells in FBS, and (2) purity of culture lines. Cell expansion required culturing on a FBS medium. For an estimated 10% to 11% of the population, this is a potential allergen. New techniques to culture and expand cells in one's own blood and also in a human platelet lysate extract eliminates this problem. Initial studies seem to indicate that human platelet lysate cytokines may actually enhance both expansion rate for stem cells and their clinical efficacy. Regarding purity of cell cultures, it has been shown that there is functional heterogeneity among mesenchymal stromal cells (MSCs). Whether these differences in MSC behavior are due to the actions of different MSC subpopulations or the effects of the tissue microenvironment on cell activity remains unknown. MSCs are heterogeneous with subpopulations of both proangiogenic and proadipogenic MSCs. There is ongoing research investigating the use of artificial niches to direct differentiation of MSCs into keratinocytes, cardio-myocytes, osteoblasts, and other cells. Future stem cell research needs to focus on answering 3 key questions: (1) What subpopulations of stem cells exist? (2) What are the parameters that define the stem cell niche? (3) What potential protumorigenic and antitumorigenic properties of stem cells can best be titrated to maximize the benefit and potential of using stem cells in reconstructive and aesthetic surgery?

Presently, ASCs appear to be the stem cells used most frequently in aesthetic and soft tissue reconstructive procedures. What are the ongoing concerns regarding ASCs in the clinical setting that need to be addressed with future research efforts? (1) ASCs prepared from human liposuction aspirate from different studies exhibit differences in purity and molecular phenotype. Many studies show that cell preparations likely contain heterogeneous populations of cells, which makes it uncertain whether the ASCs themselves are actually responsible for the observed effects. (2) Immunologic and angiogenic properties of ASCs raises questions regarding the relationship of the cells with promoting cancer. There are several contrary studies that have been published: some reports demonstrating that ASCs could promote tumor growth and other studies supporting that ASCs can have a tumor suppressive effect. Answers to the question remain unknown and further studies are necessary.

FUTURE TRENDS

Because of the volume of research compared with other cellular therapies, the impressive clinical outcomes reported in many studies, and because they are easy to obtain with minimal morbidity, ASCs appear to be the focus of most research efforts and clinical studies for cellular therapies in the aesthetic realm. Adipose tissue is currently recognized as an accessible and abundant source for adult stem cells that are suitable for tissue engineering and regenerative medicine applications. The importance of adipose tissue in future advanced cellular therapies is bolstered by the fact that adipose tissue can be cryopreserved with resultant viability of ASCs obtained from the preserved tissue. Studies have shown that adipose tissue frozen at −80°C exhibited a cellular viability of 87% after more than 1 year of cryopreservation.[146]

This opens the door to patients undergoing elective aesthetic procedures requesting that their adipose tissue be harvested and tissue banked, similar to the cryopreservation of infant cord blood and the banking of extracted wisdom teeth by oral surgeons for the preservation of dental derived stem cells. This is based on the premise that the discovery of iPSCs and their potential to function in a capacity similar to that of ESCs, will enable patients who lost the opportunity to have their cord blood preserved as newborns to take advantage of this "second chance" and have tissue preserved for therapeutic and regenerative treatments that are yet to be discovered.[1]

Although there have been significant advances made in the use of ASCs in tissue engineering, there are 2 main obstacles that continue to hinder the progress of tissue engineering: neovascularization and matrix scaffold. Biologic structures larger than 200 μm in diameter require a vascular system for nutritional support. A limited number of materials are available that can serve as scaffold that can foster tissue in growth. Innovative synthetic materials, such as polypeptides or novel biodegradable polymers, are needed that will control tissue topology and have surface modifications to stimulate cell attachment, differentiation, and growth.[1,108] The delivery of growth factors and chemical substances to guide tissue formation from stem cells encapsulated in biocompatible polymer scaffolds holds great promise for significant advances in aesthetic surgery.

Cellular therapies and tissue engineering are still in their infancy, and additional basic science and preclinical studies are needed before cosmetic and reconstructive surgical applications can be routinely undertaken and satisfactory levels of patient safety achieved.[3] However, significant advances continue to be made in the cellular therapies and tissue injury arenas. Innovations on the horizon include the following: development of xeno-free and enzyme-free culturing and manufacturing capabilities and cellular therapies derived from specific cell niches such as skin basal cell layer, hair bulb, and body tissues. All are exciting research areas that hold great promise.

From a historical perspective, new and emerging therapies and technologies have usually been met with skepticism, even those that have later become mainstay clinical therapies. In the late 1960s, a South Carolina surgeon was widely criticized for using a gastric bypass surgical technique for weight control. Today, that same therapy is viewed as the most effective treatment for morbid obesity and is the recommended treatment for those with a body mass index of 40 or higher. Using fecal implants to treat *Clostridium difficile* certainly was met with significant skepticism and was considered "over the top" when first proposed. Today, fecal microbiota transplant is considered a main line treatment, and pharmaceutical companies have invested millions of dollars in the development of fecal bacteriotherapy. It is important that as physician scientists, we keep an open mind, maintain an evidence-based perspective, and hold the safety of our patients as paramount importance.

REFERENCES

1. Beeson W, Woods E, Agha R. Tissue engineering, regenerative medicine, and rejuvenation in 2010: the role of adipose-derived stem cells. Facial Plast Surg 2011;27(4):378–87.
2. Zuk PA, Zhu M, Ashjian P, et al. Human adipose tissue is a source of multipotent stem cells. Mol Biol Cell 2002;13(12):4279–95.
3. Zuk PA. The adipose-derived stem cell: looking back and looking ahead. Mol Biol Cell 2010; 21(11):1783–7.

4. Mizuno H. Adipose-derived stem cells for tissue repair and regeneration: ten years of research and a literature review. J Nippon Med Sch 2009; 76(2):56–66.

5. Pittenger MF, Mackay AM, Beck SC, et al. Multilineage potential of adult human mesenchymal stem cells. Science 1999;284(5411):143–7.

6. Takahashi K, Tanabe K, Ohnuki M, et al. Induction of pluripotent stem cells from adult human fibroblasts by defined factors. Cell 2007;131(5):861–72.

7. Camara DA, Mambelli LI, Porcacchia AS, et al. Advances and challenges on cancer cells reprogramming using induced pluripotent stem cells technologies. J Cancer 2016;7(15):2296–303.

8. Gratama J, Kvalheim G, Orfao A. Standardization of cell analysis methods in clinical cellular therapy programs: a challenge for ISCT. Cytotherapy 2006; 8(6):528–9.

9. Bourin P, Bunnell BA, Casteilla L, et al. Stromal cells from the adipose tissue-derived stromal vascular fraction and culture expanded adipose tissue-derived stromal/stem cells: a joint statement of the International Federation for Adipose Therapeutics and Science (IFATS) and the International Society for Cellular Therapy (ISCT). Cytotherapy 2013;15(6):641–8.

10. Abbott S, Mackay G, Durdy M, et al. Twenty years of the International Society for Cellular Therapies: the past, present and future of cellular therapy clinical development. Cytotherapy 2014;16(4 Suppl): S112–9.

11. Gaur M, Dobke M, Lunyak VV. Mesenchymal stem cells from adipose tissue in clinical applications for dermatological indications and skin aging. Int J Mol Sci 2017;18(1) [pii:E208].

12. Izadpanah R, Trygg C, Patel B, et al. Biologic properties of mesenchymal stem cells derived from bone marrow and adipose tissue. J Cell Biochem 2006;99(5):1285–97.

13. Watson D, Keller GS, Lacombe V, et al. Autologous fibroblasts for treatment of facial rhytids and dermal depressions. A pilot study. Arch Facial Plast Surg 1999;1(3):165–70.

14. Mizuno H, Itoi Y, Kawahara S, et al. In vivo adipose tissue regeneration by adipose-derived stromal cells isolated from GFP transgenic mice. Cells Tissues Organs 2008;187(3):177–85.

15. Zuk PA, Zhu M, Mizuno H, et al. Multilineage cells from human adipose tissue: implications for cell-based therapies. Tissue Eng 2001;7(2):211–28.

16. Tobita M, Uysal AC, Ogawa R, et al. Periodontal tissue regeneration with adipose-derived stem cells. Tissue Eng Part A 2008;14(6):945–53.

17. Gimble JM. Adipose tissue-derived therapeutics. Expert Opin Biol Ther 2003;3(5):705–13.

18. Zouboulis CC, Makrantonaki E. Clinical aspects and molecular diagnostics of skin aging. Clin Dermatol 2011;29(1):3–14.

19. Zouboulis CC, Boschnakow A. Chronological ageing and photoageing of the human sebaceous gland. Clin Exp Dermatol 2001;26(7):600–7.

20. Kilroy GE, Foster SJ, Wu X, et al. Cytokine profile of human adipose-derived stem cells: expression of angiogenic, hematopoietic, and pro-inflammatory factors. J Cell Physiol 2007;212(3):702–9.

21. Cappuzzello C, Doni A, Dander E, et al. Mesenchymal stromal cell-derived PTX3 promotes wound healing via fibrin remodeling. J Invest Dermatol 2016;136(1):293–300.

22. Ozpur MA, Guneren E, Canter HI, et al. Generation of skin tissue using adipose tissue-derived stem cells. Plast Reconstr Surg 2016;137(1):134–43.

23. Barry BW. Novel mechanisms and devices to enable successful transdermal drug delivery. Eur J Pharm Sci 2001;14(2):101–14.

24. Elias PM, Friend DS. The permeability barrier in mammalian epidermis. J Cell Biol 1975;65(1):180–91.

25. Nemes Z, Steinert PM. Bricks and mortar of the epidermal barrier. Exp Mol Med 1999;31(1):5–19.

26. Foldvari M. Non-invasive administration of drugs through the skin: challenges in delivery system design. Pharm Sci Technolo Today 2000;3(12): 417–25.

27. Bouwstra JA, Ponec M. The skin barrier in healthy and diseased state. Biochim Biophys Acta 2006; 1758(12):2080–95.

28. Mesa KR, Rompolas P, Zito G, et al. Niche-induced cell death and epithelial phagocytosis regulate hair follicle stem cell pool. Nature 2015;522(7554):94–7.

29. Blanpain C, Fuchs E. Epidermal homeostasis: a balancing act of stem cells in the skin. Nat Rev Mol Cell Biol 2009;10(3):207–17.

30. Niu P, Smagul A, Wang L, et al. Transcriptional profiling of interleukin-2-primed human adipose derived mesenchymal stem cells revealed dramatic changes in stem cells response imposed by replicative senescence. Oncotarget 2015; 6(20):17938–57.

31. Schmidt BA, Horsley V. Intradermal adipocytes mediate fibroblast recruitment during skin wound healing. Development 2013;140(7):1517–27.

32. Kato J, Kamiya H, Himeno T, et al. Mesenchymal stem cells ameliorate impaired wound healing through enhancing keratinocyte functions in diabetic foot ulcerations on the plantar skin of rats. J Diabetes Complications 2014;28(5):588–95.

33. Kemp MG, Spandau DF, Simman R, et al. Insulin-like growth factor 1 receptor signaling is required for optimal ATR-CHK1 kinase signaling in ultraviolet B (UVB)-irradiated human keratinocytes. J Biol Chem 2017;292(4):1231–9.

34. Kemp MG, Spandau DF, Travers JB. Impact of age and insulin-like growth factor-1 on DNA damage responses in UV-irradiated human skin. Molecules 2017;22(3) [pii:E356].

35. Krbanjevic A, Travers JB, Spandau DF. How wounding via lasers has potential photocarcinogenic preventative effects via dermal remodeling. Curr Dermatol Rep 2016;5(3):222–7.

36. Lewis DA, Travers JB, Spandau DF. A new paradigm for the role of aging in the development of skin cancer. J Invest Dermatol 2009;129(3): 787–91.

37. Cao Y, Sun Z, Liao L, et al. Human adipose tissue-derived stem cells differentiate into endothelial cells in vitro and improve postnatal neovascularization in vivo. Biochem Biophys Res Commun 2005; 332(2):370–9.

38. Gimble JM, Guilak F, Bunnell BA. Clinical and preclinical translation of cell-based therapies using adipose tissue-derived cells. Stem Cell Res Ther 2010;1(2):19.

39. Gimble JM, Floyd ZE, Bunnell BA. The 4th dimension and adult stem cells: can timing be everything? J Cell Biochem 2009;107(4):569–78.

40. Waller JM, Maibach HI. Age and skin structure and function, a quantitative approach (I): blood flow, pH, thickness, and ultrasound echogenicity. Skin Res Technol 2005;11(4):221–35.

41. Farage MA, Miller KW, Elsner P, et al. Functional and physiological characteristics of the aging skin. Aging Clin Exp Res 2008;20(3):195–200.

42. Oriba HA, Bucks DA, Maibach HI. Percutaneous absorption of hydrocortisone and testosterone on the vulva and forearm: effect of the menopause and site. Br J Dermatol 1996;134(2):229–33.

43. Duncan KO, Leffell DJ. Preoperative assessment of the elderly patient. Dermatol Clin 1997;15(4): 583–93.

44. Makrantonaki E, Zouboulis CC. Molecular mechanisms of skin aging: state of the art. Ann N Y Acad Sci 2007;1119:40–50.

45. Gragnani A, Cezillo MV, da Silva ID, et al. Gene expression profile of cytokines and receptors of inflammation from cultured keratinocytes of burned patients. Burns 2014;40(5):947–56.

46. Adachi T, Kobayashi T, Sugihara E, et al. Hair follicle-derived IL-7 and IL-15 mediate skin-resident memory T cell homeostasis and lymphoma. Nat Med 2015;21(11):1272–9.

47. Knipper JA, Willenborg S, Brinckmann J, et al. Interleukin-4 receptor alpha signaling in myeloid cells controls collagen fibril assembly in skin repair. Immunity 2015;43(4):803–16.

48. Crane JD, MacNeil LG, Lally JS, et al. Exercise-stimulated interleukin-15 is controlled by AMPK and regulates skin metabolism and aging. Aging Cell 2015;14(4):625–34.

49. Kim DW, Jeon BJ, Hwang NH, et al. Adipose-derived stem cells inhibit epidermal melanocytes through an interleukin-6-mediated mechanism. Plast Reconstr Surg 2014;134(3):470–80.

50. Noordam R, Gunn DA, Tomlin CC, et al. Serum insulin-like growth factor 1 and facial ageing: high levels associate with reduced skin wrinkling in a cross-sectional study. Br J Dermatol 2013;168(3): 533–8.

51. Ezure T, Amano S. Adiponectin and leptin upregulate extracellular matrix production by dermal fibroblasts. BioFactors 2007;31(3–4):229–36.

52. Tadokoro S, Ide S, Tokuyama R, et al. Leptin promotes wound healing in the skin. PLoS One 2015; 10(3):e0121242.

53. Zhu M, Zhou Z, Chen Y, et al. Supplementation of fat grafts with adipose-derived regenerative cells improves long-term graft retention. Ann Plast Surg 2010;64(2):222–8.

54. Zhu Y, Liu T, Song K, et al. Collagen-chitosan polymer as a scaffold for the proliferation of human adipose tissue-derived stem cells. J Mater Sci Mater Med 2009;20(3):799–808.

55. Moseley TA, Zhu M, Hedrick MH. Adipose-derived stem and progenitor cells as fillers in plastic and reconstructive surgery. Plast Reconstr Surg 2006; 118(3 Suppl):121s–8s.

56. Altman AM, Abdul Khalek FJ, Seidensticker M, et al. Human tissue-resident stem cells combined with hyaluronic acid gel provide fibrovascular-integrated soft-tissue augmentation in a murine photoaged skin model. Plast Reconstr Surg 2010; 125(1):63–73.

57. Stillaert FB, Di Bartolo C, Hunt JA, et al. Human clinical experience with adipose precursor cells seeded on hyaluronic acid-based spongy scaffolds. Biomaterials 2008;29(29):3953–9.

58. Chung HJ, Jung JS, Park TG. Fabrication of adipose-derived mesenchymal stem cell aggregates using biodegradable porous microspheres for injectable adipose tissue regeneration. J Biomater Sci Polym Ed 2011;22(1–3):107–22.

59. Woo YI, Park BJ, Kim HL, et al. The biological activities of (1,3)-(1,6)-beta-d-glucan and porous electrospun PLGA membranes containing beta-glucan in human dermal fibroblasts and adipose tissue-derived stem cells. Biomed Mater 2010; 5(4):044109.

60. Tholpady SS, Llull R, Ogle RC, et al. Adipose tissue: stem cells and beyond. Clin Plast Surg 2006; 33(1):55–62, vi.

61. Yoshimura K, Suga H, Eto H. Adipose-derived stem/progenitor cells: roles in adipose tissue remodeling and potential use for soft tissue augmentation. Regen Med 2009;4(2):265–73.

62. Kapur SK, Dos-Anjos Vilaboa S, Llull R, et al. Adipose tissue and stem/progenitor cells: discovery and development. Clin Plast Surg 2015;42(2):155–67.

63. Hassan WU, Greiser U, Wang W. Role of adipose-derived stem cells in wound healing. Wound Repair Regen 2014;22(3):313–25.

64. Conde-Green A, Kotamarti VS, Sherman LS, et al. Shift toward mechanical isolation of adipose-derived stromal vascular fraction: review of upcoming techniques. Plast Reconstr Surg Glob Open 2016;4(9):e1017.

65. Negenborn VL, Groen JW, Smit JM, et al. The use of autologous fat grafting for treatment of scar tissue and scar-related conditions: a systematic review. Plast Surg Nurs 2016;36(3):131–43.

66. Shridharani SM, Broyles JM, Matarasso A. Liposuction devices: technology update. Med Devices (Auckl) 2014;7:241–51.

67. Peters EM, Liotiri S, Bodo E, et al. Probing the effects of stress mediators on the human hair follicle: substance P holds central position. Am J Pathol 2007;171(6):1872–86.

68. Banyard DA, Salibian AA, Widgerow AD, et al. Implications for human adipose-derived stem cells in plastic surgery. J Cell Mol Med 2015;19(1):21–30.

69. Cleveland EC, Albano NJ, Hazen A. Roll, spin, wash, or filter? Processing of lipoaspirate for autologous fat grafting: an updated, evidence-based review of the literature. Plast Reconstr Surg 2015;136(4):706–13.

70. Francis MP, Sachs PC, Elmore LW, et al. Isolating adipose-derived mesenchymal stem cells from lipoaspirate blood and saline fraction. Organogenesis 2010;6(1):11–4.

71. Hanke A, Prantl L, Wenzel C, et al. Semi-automated extraction and characterization of stromal vascular fraction using a new medical device. Clin Hemorheol Microcirc 2016;64(3):403–12.

72. Grasys J, Kim BS, Pallua N. Content of soluble factors and characteristics of stromal vascular fraction cells in lipoaspirates from different subcutaneous adipose tissue depots. Aesthet Surg J 2016; 36(7):831–41.

73. Kakagia D, Pallua N. Autologous fat grafting: in search of the optimal technique. Surg Innov 2014; 21(3):327–36.

74. Strong AL, Cederna PS, Rubin JP, et al. The current state of fat grafting: a review of harvesting, processing, and injection techniques. Plast Reconstr Surg 2015;136(4):897–912.

75. Strioga M, Viswanathan S, Darinskas A, et al. Same or not the same? Comparison of adipose tissue-derived versus bone marrow-derived mesenchymal stem and stromal cells. Stem Cells Dev 2012;21(14):2724–52.

76. Melief SM, Schrama E, Brugman MH, et al. Multipotent stromal cells induce human regulatory T cells through a novel pathway involving skewing of monocytes toward anti-inflammatory macrophages. Stem cells 2013;31(9):1980–91.

77. Li CY, Wu XY, Tong JB, et al. Comparative analysis of human mesenchymal stem cells from bone marrow and adipose tissue under xeno-free conditions for cell therapy. Stem Cell Res Ther 2015;6:55.

78. Toyserkani NM, Christensen ML, Sheikh SP, et al. Adipose-derived stem cells: new treatment for wound healing? Ann Plast Surg 2015;75(1):117–23.

79. Stessuk T, Puzzi MB, Chaim EA, et al. Platelet-rich plasma (PRP) and adipose-derived mesenchymal stem cells: stimulatory effects on proliferation and migration of fibroblasts and keratinocytes in vitro. Arch Dermatol Res 2016;308(7):511–20.

80. Son WC, Yun JW, Kim BH. Adipose-derived mesenchymal stem cells reduce MMP-1 expression in UV-irradiated human dermal fibroblasts: therapeutic potential in skin wrinkling. Biosci Biotechnol Biochem 2015;79(6):919–25.

81. Hocking AM, Gibran NS. Mesenchymal stem cells: paracrine signaling and differentiation during cutaneous wound repair. Exp Cell Res 2010;316(14): 2213–9.

82. Lopez MF, Niu P, Wang L, et al. Opposing activities of oncogenic MIR17HG and tumor suppressive MIR100HG clusters and their gene targets regulate replicative senescence in human adult stem cells. NPJ Aging Mech Dis 2017;3:7.

83. Tollervey JR, Lunyak VV. Adult stem cells: simply a tool for regenerative medicine or an additional piece in the puzzle of human aging? Cell Cycle 2011;10(24):4173–6.

84. Bhandari DR, Seo KW, Sun B, et al. The simplest method for in vitro beta-cell production from human adult stem cells. Differentiation 2011;82(3):144–52.

85. Gruber HE, Somayaji S, Riley F, et al. Human adipose-derived mesenchymal stem cells: serial passaging, doubling time and cell senescence. Biotech Histochem 2012;87(4):303–11.

86. Jun HS, Dao LT, Pyun JC, et al. Effect of cell senescence on the impedance measurement of adipose tissue-derived stem cells. Enzyme Microb Technol 2013;53(5):302–6.

87. von Mering C, Jensen LJ, Snel B, et al. STRING: known and predicted protein-protein associations, integrated and transferred across organisms. Nucleic Acids Res 2005;33(Database issue):D433–7.

88. Jeyapalan JC, Sedivy JM. Cellular senescence and organismal aging. Mech Ageing Dev 2008; 129(7–8):467–74.

89. Song SY, Jung JE, Jeon YR, et al. Determination of adipose-derived stem cell application on photoaged fibroblasts, based on paracrine function. Cytotherapy 2011;13(3):378–84.

90. Park BS, Jang KA, Sung JH, et al. Adipose-derived stem cells and their secretory factors as a promising therapy for skin aging. Dermatol Surg 2008; 34(10):1323–6.

91. Mehta RC, Fitzpatrick RE. Endogenous growth factors as cosmeceuticals. Dermatol Ther 2007;20(5): 350–9.

92. Kim SG, Kim EY, Kim YJ, et al. The efficacy and safety of ablative fractional resurfacing using a 2,940-Nm Er:YAG laser for traumatic scars in the early posttraumatic period. Arch Plast Surg 2012; 39(3):232–7.

93. Issler-Fisher AC, Waibel JS, Donelan MB. Laser modulation of hypertrophic scars: technique and practice. Clin Plast Surg 2017;44(4):757–66.

94. Waibel JS, Rudnick A. Laser-assisted delivery to treat facial scars. Facial Plast Surg Clin North Am 2017;25(1):105–17.

95. Waibel JS, Rudnick A, Shagalov DR, et al. Update of ablative fractionated lasers to enhance cutaneous topical drug delivery. Adv Ther 2017;34(8):1840–9.

96. Waibel JS, Rudnick AC, Wulkan AJ, et al. The diagnostic role of optical coherence tomography (OCT) in measuring the depth of burn and traumatic scars for more accurate laser dosimetry: pilot study. J Drugs Dermatol 2016;15(11):1375–80.

97. Waibel JS, Wulkan AJ, Shumaker PR. Treatment of hypertrophic scars using laser and laser assisted corticosteroid delivery. Lasers Surg Med 2013; 45(3):135–40.

98. Kim WS, Park BS, Park SH, et al. Antiwrinkle effect of adipose-derived stem cell: activation of dermal fibroblast by secretory factors. J Dermatol Sci 2009;53(2):96–102.

99. Brohem CA, de Carvalho CM, Radoski CL, et al. Comparison between fibroblasts and mesenchymal stem cells derived from dermal and adipose tissue. Int J Cosmet Sci 2013;35(5):448–57.

100. Fabi S, Sundaram H. The potential of topical and injectable growth factors and cytokines for skin rejuvenation. Facial Plast Surg 2014;30(2):157–71.

101. Lee HJ, Lee EG, Kang S, et al. Efficacy of microneedling plus human stem cell conditioned medium for skin rejuvenation: a randomized, controlled, blinded split-face study. Ann Dermatol 2014;26(5):584–91.

102. Sasaki GH. Response to commentaries on "microneedling depth penetration, presence of pigment particles, and fluorescein-stained platelets: clinical usage for aesthetic concerns.". Aesthet Surg J 2017;37(5):NP60–1.

103. Sasaki GH. Micro-needling depth penetration, presence of pigment particles, and fluorescein-stained platelets: clinical usage for aesthetic concerns. Aesthet Surg J 2017;37(1):71–83.

104. Hussain M, Phelps R, Goldberg DJ. Clinical, histologic, and ultrastructural changes after use of human growth factor and cytokine skin cream for the treatment of skin rejuvenation. J Cosmet Laser Ther 2008;10(2):104–9.

105. Sundaram H, Mehta RC, Norine JA, et al. Topically applied physiologically balanced growth factors: a new paradigm of skin rejuvenation. J Drugs Dermatol 2009;8(5 Suppl Skin Rejuenation):4–13.

106. Fitzpatrick RE, Rostan EF. Reversal of photodamage with topical growth factors: a pilot study. J Cosmet Laser Ther 2003;5(1):25–34.

107. Sterodimas A, De Faria J, Correa WE, et al. Tissue engineering in plastic surgery: an up-to-date review of the current literature. Ann Plast Surg 2009;62(1):97–103.

108. Sterodimas A, de Faria J, Nicaretta B, et al. Cell-assisted lipotransfer. Aesthet Surg J 2010;30(1): 78–81.

109. Garcia-Olmo D, Garcia-Arranz M, Herreros D. Expanded adipose-derived stem cells for the treatment of complex perianal fistula including Crohn's disease. Expert Opin Biol Ther 2008;8(9):1417–23.

110. Yoshimura K, Sato K, Aoi N, et al. Cell-assisted lipotransfer for facial lipoatrophy: efficacy of clinical use of adipose-derived stem cells. Dermatol Surg 2008;34(9):1178–85.

111. Rubin JP, Marra KG. Soft tissue reconstruction. Methods Mol Biol 2011;702:395–400.

112. Rubin JP, Marra KG. Commentary. Cell-assisted lipotransfer (CAL). Aesthet Surg J 2010;30(1):82.

113. Matsumoto D, Sato K, Gonda K, et al. Cell-assisted lipotransfer: supportive use of human adipose-derived cells for soft tissue augmentation with lipoinjection. Tissue Eng 2006;12(12):3375–82.

114. Yoshimura K, Sato K, Aoi N, et al. Cell-assisted lipotransfer for cosmetic breast augmentation: supportive use of adipose-derived stem/stromal cells. Aesthetic Plast Surg 2008;32(1):48–55 [discussion: 6–7].

115. Tanikawa DY, Aguena M, Bueno DF, et al. Fat grafts supplemented with adipose-derived stromal cells in the rehabilitation of patients with craniofacial microsomia. Plast Reconstr Surg 2013;132(1): 141–52.

116. Kolle SF, Fischer-Nielsen A, Mathiasen AB, et al. Enrichment of autologous fat grafts with ex-vivo expanded adipose tissue-derived stem cells for graft survival: a randomised placebo-controlled trial. Lancet 2013;382(9898):1113–20.

117. Garza RM, Paik KJ, Chung MT, et al. Studies in fat grafting: part III. Fat grafting irradiated tissue–improved skin quality and decreased fat graft retention. Plast Reconstr Surg 2014;134(2):249–57.

118. Ansorge H, Garza JR, McCormack MC, et al. Autologous fat processing via the Revolve system: quality and quantity of fat retention evaluated in an animal model. Aesthet Surg J 2014;34(3):438–47.

119. Suga H, Eto H, Aoi N, et al. Adipose tissue remodeling under ischemia: death of adipocytes and activation of stem/progenitor cells. Plast Reconstr Surg 2010;126(6):1911–23.

120. Kato H, Araki J, Doi K, et al. Normobaric hyperoxygenation enhances initial survival, regeneration, and final retention in fat grafting. Plast Reconstr Surg 2014;134(5):951–9.

121. Pan Z, Duan P, Liu X, et al. Effect of porosities of bilayered porous scaffolds on spontaneous osteochondral repair in cartilage tissue engineering. Regen Biomater 2015;2(1):9–19.

122. Lu W, Si YI, Ding J, et al. Mesenchymal stem cells attenuate acute ischemia-reperfusion injury in a rat model. Exp Ther Med 2015;10(6):2131–7.

123. van Harmelen V, Skurk T, Hauner H. Primary culture and differentiation of human adipocyte precursor cells. Methods Mol Med 2005;107:125–35.

124. Yoshimura K, Asano Y, Aoi N, et al. Progenitor-enriched adipose tissue transplantation as rescue for breast implant complications. Breast J 2010; 16(2):169–75.

125. Paik KJ, Zielins ER, Atashroo DA, et al. Studies in fat grafting: part V. Cell-assisted lipotransfer to enhance fat graft retention is dose dependent. Plast Reconstr Surg 2015;136(1):67–75.

126. Levi B, Nelson ER, Li S, et al. Dura mater stimulates human adipose-derived stromal cells to undergo bone formation in mouse calvarial defects. Stem cells 2011;29(8):1241–55.

127. Levi B, James AW, Nelson ER, et al. Studies in adipose-derived stromal cells: migration and participation in repair of cranial injury after systemic injection. Plast Reconstr Surg 2011;127(3): 1130–40.

128. Levi B, Hyun JS, Nelson ER, et al. Nonintegrating knockdown and customized scaffold design enhances human adipose-derived stem cells in skeletal repair. Stem cells 2011;29(12):2018–29.

129. Yeh HY, Lin TY, Lin CH, et al. Neocartilage formation from mesenchymal stem cells grown in type II collagen-hyaluronan composite scaffolds. Differentiation 2013;86(4–5):171–83.

130. Jeong IH, Shetty AA, Kim SJ, et al. Autologous collagen-induced chondrogenesis using fibrin and atelocollagen mixture. Cells Tissues Organs 2013;198(4):278–88.

131. Scott MA, Nguyen VT, Levi B, et al. Current methods of adipogenic differentiation of mesenchymal stem cells. Stem Cells Dev 2011;20(10): 1793–804.

132. Memon B, Karam M, Al-Khawaga S, et al. Enhanced differentiation of human pluripotent stem cells into pancreatic progenitors co-expressing PDX1 and NKX6.1. Stem Cell Res Ther 2018;9(1):15.

133. Sivan U, Jayakumar K, Krishnan LK. Matrix-directed differentiation of human adipose-derived mesenchymal stem cells to dermal-like fibroblasts that produce extracellular matrix. J Tissue Eng Regen Med 2016;10(10):E546–58.

134. Sivan U, Jayakumar K, Krishnan LK. Constitution of fibrin-based niche for in vitro differentiation of adipose-derived mesenchymal stem cells to keratinocytes. Biores Open Access 2014;3(6): 339–47.

135. Fullgrabe A, Joost S, Are A, et al. Dynamics of Lgr6(+) progenitor cells in the hair follicle, sebaceous gland, and interfollicular epidermis. Stem Cell Reports 2015;5(5):843–55.

136. Rubio D, Garcia-Castro J, Martin MC, et al. Spontaneous human adult stem cell transformation. Cancer Res 2005;65(8):3035–9.

137. Schweizer R, Tsuji W, Gorantla VS, et al. The role of adipose-derived stem cells in breast cancer progression and metastasis. Stem Cells Int 2015 2015;120949.

138. Ning H, Yang F, Jiang M, et al. The correlation between cotransplantation of mesenchymal stem cells and higher recurrence rate in hematologic malignancy patients: outcome of a pilot clinical study. Leukemia 2008;22(3):593–9.

139. Kucerova L, Matuskova M, Hlubinova K, et al. Tumor cell behaviour modulation by mesenchymal stromal cells. Mol Cancer 2010;9:129.

140. Mishra PJ, Mishra PJ, Humeniuk R, et al. Carcinoma-associated fibroblast-like differentiation of human mesenchymal stem cells. Cancer Res 2008;68(11):4331–9.

141. Karnoub AE, Dash AB, Vo AP, et al. Mesenchymal stem cells within tumour stroma promote breast cancer metastasis. Nature 2007;449(7162):557–63.

142. Mendicino M, Bailey AM, Wonnacott K, et al. MSC-based product characterization for clinical trials: an FDA perspective. Cell Stem Cell 2014;14(2):141–5.

143. Gir P, Oni G, Brown SA, et al. Human adipose stem cells: current clinical applications. Plast Reconstr Surg 2012;129(6):1277–90.

144. Kellathur SN, Lou HX. Cell and tissue therapy regulation: worldwide status and harmonization. Biologicals 2012;40(3):222–4.

145. Hayakawa T, Harris I, Joung J, et al. Report of the international regulatory forum on human cell therapy and gene therapy products. Biologicals 2016;44(5):467–79.

146. Lee JE, Kim I, Kim M. Adipogenic differentiation of human adipose tissue-derived stem cells obtained from cryopreserved adipose aspirates. Dermatol Surg 2010;36(7):1078–83.

UNITED STATES POSTAL SERVICE ®

Statement of Ownership, Management, and Circulation (All Periodicals Publications Except Requester Publications)

1. Publication Title	2. Publication Number	3. Filing Date
FACIAL PLASTIC SURGERY CLINICS OF NORTH AMERICA	013 – 122	9/18/2018

4. Issue Frequency	5. Number of Issues Published Annually	6. Annual Subscription Price
FEB, MAY, AUG, NOV	4	$398.00

7. Complete Mailing Address of Known Office of Publication (Not printer) (Street, city, county, state, and ZIP+4®)

ELSEVIER INC.
230 Park Avenue, Suite 800
New York, NY 10169

Contact Person
STEPHEN R. BUSHING

Telephone (Include area code)
215-239-3688

8. Complete Mailing Address of Headquarters or General Business Office of Publisher (Not printer)

ELSEVIER INC.
230 Park Avenue, Suite 800
New York, NY 10169

9. Full Names and Complete Mailing Addresses of Publisher, Editor, and Managing Editor (Do not leave blank)

Publisher (Name and complete mailing address)

TAYLOR E BALL, ELSEVIER INC.
1600 JOHN F KENNEDY BLVD. SUITE 1800
PHILADELPHIA, PA 19103-2899

Editor (Name and complete mailing address)

JESSICA MCCOOL, ELSEVIER INC.
1600 JOHN F KENNEDY BLVD. SUITE 1800
PHILADELPHIA, PA 19103-2899

Managing Editor (Name and complete mailing address)

PATRICK MANLEY, ELSEVIER INC.
1600 JOHN F KENNEDY BLVD. SUITE 1800
PHILADELPHIA, PA 19103-2899

10. Owner (Do not leave blank. If the publication is owned by a corporation, give the name and address of the corporation immediately followed by the names and addresses of all stockholders owning or holding 1 percent or more of the total amount of stock. If not owned by a corporation, give the names and addresses of the individual owners. If owned by a partnership or other unincorporated firm, give its name and address as well as those of each individual owner. If the publication is published by a nonprofit organization, give its name and address.)

Full Name	Complete Mailing Address
WHOLLY OWNED SUBSIDIARY OF REED/ELSEVIER, US HOLDINGS	1600 JOHN F KENNEDY BLVD, SUITE 1800 PHILADELPHIA, PA 19103-2899

11. Known Bondholders, Mortgagees, and Other Security Holders Owning or Holding 1 Percent or More of Total Amount of Bonds, Mortgages, or Other Securities. If none, check box. → ☐ None

Full Name	Complete Mailing Address
N/A	

12. Tax Status (For completion by nonprofit organizations authorized to mail at nonprofit rates) (Check one)
The purpose, function, and nonprofit status of this organization and the exempt status for federal income tax purposes:
☒ Has Not Changed During Preceding 12 Months
☐ Has Changed During Preceding 12 Months (Publisher must submit explanation of change with this statement)

PS Form **3526**, July 2014 [Page 1 of 4 (see instructions page 4)]   PSN: 7530-01-000-9931   PRIVACY NOTICE: See our privacy policy on www.usps.com.

---

13. Publication Title	14. Issue Date for Circulation Data Below
FACIAL PLASTIC SURGERY CLINICS OF NORTH AMERICA	MAY 2018

15. Extent and Nature of Circulation			Average No. Copies Each Issue During Preceding 12 Months	No. Copies of Single Issue Published Nearest to Filing Date
a. Total Number of Copies (Net press run)			175	266
b. Paid Circulation (By Mail and Outside the Mail)	(1)	Mailed Outside-County Paid Subscriptions Stated on PS Form 3541 (Include paid distribution above nominal rate, advertiser's proof copies, and exchange copies)	101	156
	(2)	Mailed In-County Paid Subscriptions Stated on PS Form 3541 (Include paid distribution above nominal rate, advertiser's proof copies, and exchange copies)	0	0
	(3)	Paid Distribution Outside the Mails Including Sales Through Dealers and Carriers, Street Vendors, Counter Sales, and Other Paid Distribution Outside USPS®	17	23
	(4)	Paid Distribution by Other Classes of Mail Through the USPS (e.g., First-Class Mail®)	0	0
c. Total Paid Distribution (Sum of 15b (1), (2), (3), and (4))			118	179
d. Free or Nominal Rate Distribution (By Mail and Outside the Mail)	(1)	Free or Nominal Rate Outside-County Copies included on PS Form 3541	48	74
	(2)	Free or Nominal Rate In-County Copies Included on PS Form 3541	0	0
	(3)	Free or Nominal Rate Copies Mailed at Other Classes Through the USPS (e.g., First-Class Mail)	0	0
	(4)	Free or Nominal Rate Distribution Outside the Mail (Carriers or other means)	0	0
e. Total Free or Nominal Rate Distribution (Sum of 15d (1), (2), (3) and (4))			48	74
f. Total Distribution (Sum of 15c and 15e)			166	253
g. Copies not Distributed (See Instructions to Publishers #4 (page 83))			9	15
h. Total (Sum of 15f and g)			175	268
i. Percent Paid (15c divided by 15f times 100)			71.08%	70.75%

* If you are claiming electronic copies, go to line 16 on page 3. If you are not claiming electronic copies, skip to line 17 on page 3.

16. Electronic Copy Circulation	Average No. Copies Each Issue During Preceding 12 Months	No. Copies of Single Issue Published Nearest to Filing Date
a. Paid Electronic Copies ▲	0	0
b. Total Paid Print Copies (Line 15c) + Paid Electronic Copies (Line 16a) ▲	118	179
c. Total Print Distribution (Line 15f) + Paid Electronic Copies (Line 16a) ▲	166	253
d. Percent Paid (Both Print & Electronic Copies) (16b divided by 16c × 100) ▲	71.08%	70.75

☒ I certify that 50% of all my distributed copies (electronic and print) are paid above a nominal price.

17. Publication of Statement of Ownership

☒ If the publication is a general publication, publication of this statement is required. Will be printed in the NOVEMBER 2018 issue of this publication.   ☐ Publication not required.

18. Signature and Title of Editor, Publisher, Business Manager, or Owner

STEPHEN R. BUSHING - INVENTORY DISTRIBUTION CONTROL MANAGER

Date 9/18/2018

I certify that all information furnished on this form is true and complete. I understand that anyone who furnishes false or misleading information on this form or who omits material or information requested on the form may be subject to criminal sanctions (including fines and imprisonment) and/or civil sanctions (including civil penalties).

PS Form **3526**, July 2014 (Page 2 of 4)   PRIVACY NOTICE: See our privacy policy on www.usps.com

Printed and bound by CPI Group (UK) Ltd, Croydon, CR0 4YY

08/05/2025

01864732-0001